Management of Depression

Dr Gin Malhi and Dr Paul Bridges

The Geoffrey Knight National Unit for
Affective Disorders

The Maudsley Hospital

Denmark Hill

Camberwell

London SE5 8AZ

With a foreword by Professor Ted Dinan

Published with the assistance of an
educational grant from

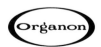

© Martin Dunitz 1998

First published in the United Kingdom in 1998 by:

Martin Dunitz Ltd
The Livery House
7–9 Pratt Street
London NW1 0AE

A CIP record for this book is available from the British Library.

ISBN 1-85317-702-4

Printed and bound in Italy.

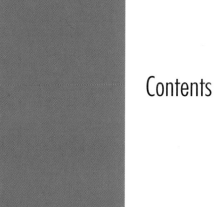

Contents

Acknowledgements

The authors would like to thank Dr Jerome Carson, Dr Anthony Davies, Dr Frank Holloway and Dr Eileen McGinley for their invaluable help.

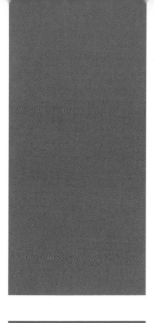

Foreword

Research into the causes and management of depression has undergone an exponential increase over the past decade, with greater acknowledgement of the fact that depression represents a major health issue and one for which far better and more acceptable pharmacological strategies are available. The consequences of undetected and untreated depression are significant from both a psychosocial and physical perspective. The risk of suicide and the impact on family life and work performance are all well recognized, together with the increasing realization that untreated or poorly treated depression may negatively influence physical health, for example increasing the risk of coronary artery disease.

Within the above context the publication of this book is to be welcomed. Whilst many valuable texts have been published on the subject, few concise yet comprehensive overviews are available. This book provides an up-to-date account of depression in terms of clinical diagnosis, aetiology and comprehensive management, together with a review of depression in specific clinical populations. The authors, Dr Bridges and Dr Malhi, are to be commended on the outcome of their work.

Dr Bridges is an international figure in the field of depression research, and an authority on the use of psychosurgery for the treatment of resistant depression, and Dr Malhi is a Senior Registrar working in the same field. Working on a book such as this is never an easy task. Striking an appropriate balance between being comprehensive yet concise is difficult to achieve. Dr Bridges and Dr Malhi have succeeded and produced a readable volume which will be valued by the target audience.

The book should have a wide readership. Those training for the MRCPsych examination will definitely find it of value, as will many general practitioners. Psychologists in training and basic scientists wishing to obtain an overview of depression will undoubtedly benefit from a read. It would be difficult to produce a more informative, user-friendly volume.

Professor Ted Dinan
Department of Psychiatry
Royal College of Surgeons in Ireland

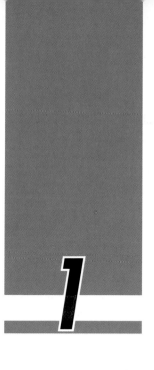

Signs and symptoms of depression

Introduction

The term depression is used in a variety of ways. In everyday language, it is commonly used to describe feelings of sadness or despondency. These feelings are part of normal emotion and may be the consequence of disappointments or failures.

As a medical term, depression can refer to a symptom, syndrome or illness. In its usual clinical context, depression denotes a disorder of mood that is distinct from normality. Qualitatively, the sustained, pervasive feelings of misery, despair and hopelessness that are characteristic of depressive illness are very different from the normal feelings of unhappiness or sadness.

Disorders involving abnormalities of mood used to be called manic-depressive but are now more often termed affective disorders. This is more accurate because only a minority of sufferers experience episodes of both mania and depression (bipolar affective disorder) and most have recurrent episodes of depression only (unipolar depression).

Defining depression involves delineating it from normality by identifying reliably its signs and symptoms, and distinguishing it from other psychiatric syndromes. The psychopathology of depression character-izes the illness and gives rise to its many presentations. Therefore, in practice, knowledge of the clinical features of depression is essential, and so these are described in detail.

Clinical features of depression

Appearance and behaviour

The typical depressed patient avoids eye-contact by averting their gaze downwards and sitting with a slumped posture, in which the head is inclined forward and the shoulders are hunched. Inspection of the face reveals vertical furrowing of the brow, down-turned corners of the mouth and a reduced rate of blinking. There is a reduction in the number of gestures and the speed at which these are made; however, in the presence of concomitant anxiety there may be an increase in move-ments with restlessness and agitation. Sometimes there is a degree of general self-neglect, reflected in poor hygiene, grooming and dress.[1]

Speech

Depressed individuals often speak slowly in a quiet, monotonous voice. In severe depression there is a paucity of words with notable pauses in conversation and long delays in responding to questions. Sponta-neous speech is noticeably absent.

Mood

The primary complaint in depression is that of low mood. However, it is important to note that not all patients who complain of being low in mood are depressed, and those who have a depressive illness may in fact present with physical symptoms, especially pain, and do not necessarily consider their mental health a problem. Depressed mood is usually described by the patient as a feeling of sadness or hope-lessness but it can also present as apathy or irritability, and so questioning should attempt to understand fully the patient's emotional state.[2]

Fatigue and lethargy

Depressed patients often report feelings of being run down and of heaviness in the limbs. They lack energy and feel exhausted all the time. Loss of energy and fatigue are characteristic symptoms of depression.

Biological symptoms of depression

When assessing mood it is also necessary to consider the biological (sometimes called somatic, endogenous, melancholic, vegetative) symptoms of depression shown in *Table 1.1*, as these have particular clinical significance. Occasionally they are grouped together as a syndrome and, because of their importance, they are discussed further.[3]

Constipation, menstrual irregularities and loss of libido are common complaints of biological depressives and although important symptoms they are often overlooked. Presence of these symptoms should prompt inquiry about mood.

Diurnal variation of mood

This is a symptom specific to biological depression. The mood of depressives is characteristically at its lowest upon waking. During the course of the day it improves and this pattern of change is described as the diurnal variation of mood. It is an important biological symptom as the clinical presentation of a patient may vary considerably according to the time of day.[4]

Table 1.1
Biological symptoms of depression.

- Reduced appetite and weight
- Early morning wakening
- Diurnal variation of mood
- Anhedonia
- Reduced libido
- Menstrual irregularities
- Constipation

Sleep

In depression, sleep disturbance is a common complaint. Initial insomnia (that is, difficulty in falling asleep) and the interruption of sleep are both changes that diminish the quality of sleep in depressives such that they often wake unrefreshed and tired even if their sleep has been of normal duration. Early morning wakening is a characteristic feature of depressive disorders, with the patient waking a few hours before their usual time, typically 4–5 am, and then being unable to resume sleep. It is at this time that depressed mood is at its lowest and the patient then often spends this extra time engaged in pessimistic and negative thoughts. Hence, the combination of early morning wakening and diurnal variation of mood increases the suicide risk.[5]

Appetite and weight

Ordinarily, in depression, there is a reduction of both appetite and weight. Typically, more than 5% of total body weight is lost over a period of a month and this is not wholly accounted for by diminished nourishment.

Anhedonia

In depressive illness the ability to experience emotion is usually constricted and often restricted to depressed mood. Occasionally, the patient may not be able to experience any emotions and this is often a distressing symptom which the patient may be unable to describe. Sometimes, the individual loses the feeling of familiarity with surroundings or self. This is called *depersonalization*, and it is characteristically an intensely unpleasant experience. The more specific loss of the capacity to feel emotion, for example the inability to cry, is termed *deaffectualization*. *Anhedonia* is a component of this and describes the complete inability to enjoy life or gain pleasure from activities that would normally provide gratification, such as food, hobbies, company of others and sex. Clinically, it is an important symptom as it plays a central role in the diagnosis and management of depression.[6]

Reversed biological symptoms

In some cases of depression there is an increase in appetite and weight, combined with increased sleep. These are described as 'reversed biological symptoms' and are thought to be associated with 'atypical depression' in which the accompanying depressed mood is described as reactive *(Chapter 2)*.

Suicidality

It is essential to ask all depressed patients about thoughts concerning suicide while bearing in mind that even upon direct inquiry not all will be forthcoming with the truth. The intensity of such ideas should be gauged by questioning the frequency of suicidal thoughts and the extent to which plans have been made. Suicide, and the assessment of risk, are discussed further in **Chapter 10**.

Anxiety

Depressed patients often experience symptoms of anxiety. However, anxiety may completely dominate the clinical picture, as in agitated depression, where the patient is restless and unable to sit or stand still, usually pacing around, unable to occupy themselves and, instead, wringing their hands. This type of presentation carries a serious risk of suicide and yet the patient may not acknowledge or be aware of such a risk and may deny any change of mood.

The appearance of an extremely anxious person is quite distinctive. The skin is often pale and sweaty and the individual has a strained expression with a furrowed brow. Physically the person is tense, restless and occasionally tremulous. The features of anxiety fall in two groups: psychological symptoms and somatic symptoms.[7] These are listed in **Table 1.2**.

Obsessions and compulsions

Obsessional symptoms, which are also relatively common in the setting of depressive illnesses reduce the likelihood of self-harm (unlike comorbid symptoms of anxiety). They can be secondary to depression or conversely depressive symptoms can arise in the context of an obsessional disorder. Obsessional symptoms as part of a mood disorder usually subside if this is successfully treated. The characteristic feature of obsessions (thoughts, ideas, images or impulses) is that they are distressing and enter the patient's mind repeatedly in a stereotyped form. The patient tries to resist them, usually unsuccessfully, whilst acknowledging that they are their own thoughts. Compulsive acts are behaviours that have the same features as obsessions and result in useless rituals that are not inherently enjoyable and do not seem reasonable to the patient. Examples of some common obsessions are given in **Table 1.3**.[8]

Thoughts

Depression is associated with certain kinds of thoughts described variously as negative beliefs, pessimistic thoughts or depressive cognitions. Depressives have a

Psychological	Somatic
Apprehension and fear	**Cardiovascular**
• Of going mad	• Palpitations
• Of dying	• Tachycardia
• Of disaster	• Feeling of missed beats
Fearful anticipation	**Respiratory**
• Of losing control	• Breathlessness
• Of passing out	• Over-breathing
Intense inner tension	**Gastrointestinal**
• Feeling 'on edge'	• Dry mouth
• Inability to relax	• Dysphagia
• Worry	• Nausea
	• Epigastric discomfort
Irritability	• Diarrhoea
• Noise intolerance	
	Genitourinary
Distractible	• Urinary frequency
• Difficulty concentrating, hence poor memory	• Urinary urgency
	• Menstrual discomfort
	• Erectile failure
Depersonalization	
• Feeling unreal	**Muscular Tension**
	• Headache
	• Tremor / trembling

Table 1.2
Features of anxiety.

negative view of the world concerning the past, present and future which colours their thinking and contributes to their illness. They ruminate about losses, in particular deaths, and often have feelings of guilt, self-reproach, helplessness and

Obsessive ruminations	Obsessive compulsions
Repeated doubts	Repeated checking
Worry about contamination	Repeated hand washing and cleaning
A need for order or symmetry	Counting

Table 1.3
Obsessive symptoms.

hopelessness. These thoughts are associated with feelings of inadequacy and low self-esteem, prompting suicidal ideation.[9] The complex basis of such thinking is discussed later along with the various methods that can be used to treat depression by changing these patterns of thought. *(Chapter 6)*.

Psychomotor retardation

Psychomotor retardation refers to the slowing of thought that occurs in depression along with the observed reduction of movements and activity. It results in delayed verbal and behavioural responses.[10]

Delusions

Psychotic depression is usually characterized by the presence of delusions. These centre on the main themes of depression, namely, guilt, worries of ill-health (hypochondriacal), poverty and feelings of worthlessness and persecution. When very severe the patient may deny the existence of bodily parts, themselves or indeed that of the world around them ('nihilistic delusions'). The delusions are different from those of schizophrenic illnesses in that they are mood congruent and 'understandable' in the context of depression.[11]

Cognition

It is well recognized that the depressed state impairs thinking, in particular concentration and memory. Deficits in this area of functioning should not be construed as problems of an uncooperative or manipulative personality. Often the abnormalities are so subtle that the patient may not notice them and it is relatives and friends who first detect a change. Psychological testing can identify cognitive changes and help clarify the cause.

Accuracy is usually retained but speed and performance are slowed. This is particularly relevant to elderly patients in whom other aetiologies, for example dementia, may need to be excluded[12, 13] *(Chapter 9).*

Insight

The judgement and insight of a depressed patient are best assessed by reviewing the patient's recent decisions and actions and exploring their current ideas and intentions.

The ability to make judgements and the possession of insight are important as they have implications regarding treatment and self-harm. These aspects of mentation can be modified by depression to the extent that patients find it difficult to take decisions and make plans. Furthermore they may not be fully aware of the future consequences of their actions and these aspects are particularly important when considering compulsory admission to hospital or emergency treatment.

Key Points

• Depressive illness is distinct from the normal vicissitudes of mood.

• In the absence of reliable biological markers, depression is best defined clinically by description of its signs and symptoms.

• Typically, the clinical features of depressive illness include:
  1. reduced eye-contact and a slowing of movement and speech
  2. low mood that is pervasive and persistent and often accompanied by suicidal ideation
  3. the biological symptoms of depression

• Symptoms of comorbid anxiety are common and their presence or that of obsessive symptoms should prompt inquiry about mood.

• Severe depressive illnesses can present with psychotic symptoms or cognitive impairment and occasionally compromise insight.

References

1. McGuire GP. The psychiatric interview. In: Kendall RE, Zealley AK eds, *Companion to Psychiatric Studies*, 5th edn (London: Churchill Livingstone, 1993) 263–76.

2. Kendall RE. Mood (affective) disorders. In: Kendall RE, Zealley AK eds, *Companion to Psychiatric Studies*, 5th edn (London: Churchill Livingstone, 1993) 427–57.

3. Bech P. Symptoms and assessment of depression. In: Paykel ES ed, *Handbook of Affective Disorders*, 2nd edn (New York: Churchill Livingstone, 1992) 3–13.

4. Moffoot APR, O'Carroll RE, Bennie J et al. Diurnal variation of mood and neuropsychological function in major depression with melancholia. *Journal of Affective Disorders* (1994) 32: 257–69.

5. Nelson JC, Charney DS. The symptoms of major depressive illness. *American Journal of Psychiatry* (1981) 138: 1–13.

6. Sims A. *Symptoms in the Mind*, 2nd edn (London: Saunders, 1995).

7. Gelder M, Gath D, Mayou R. *Oxford Textbook of Psychiatry*, 2nd edn (Oxford: Oxford Medical Publications, 1992).

8. Marks IM. Fears, phobias and rituals. In: *Panic, Anxiety and Their Disorders* (Oxford:OUP, 1987) 423–53.

9. Kaplan HI, Sadock BJ, Grebb JA. *Synopsis of Psychiatry*, 7th edn (Baltimore MD: Williams & Wilkins, 1994).

10. Avery D, Silverman J. Psychomotor retardation and agitation in depression: relationship to age, sex and response to treatment. *Journal of Affective Disorders* (1984) 7: 67–76.

11. Hamilton M. *Fish's Clinical Psychopathology, Signs and Symptoms in Psychiatry* (Bristol: Wright, 1974).

12. Baldwin RC. Depressive illness. In: Jacoby R and Oppenheimer C eds, *Psychiatry in the Elderly* (Oxford: Oxford University Press, 1991) 676–719.

13. Sobin C, Sackheim HA. Psychomotor symptoms of depression. *American Journal of Psychiatry* (1997) 154: 4–17.

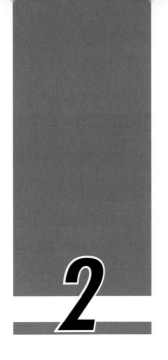

Diagnosis, classification and epidemiology

2

Diagnosis

In the absence of reliable biological markers, the diagnosis of depression remains dependent upon the recognition and classification of signs and symptoms. The criteria used to make a diagnosis vary according to purpose and application such that research criteria are usually more specific and exacting than those used in clinical practice. Consequently, there are now a variety of terms that describe groups of depressive symptoms, some of which are better defined than others. There are two major systems of classification which describe these depressive syndromes in detail and provide 'diagnostic criteria' for clinical and research purposes. The categories used to describe these syndromes are shown in **Tables 2.1**, **2.2**, and **2.3**.

ICD-10	DSM-IV
Depressive episode: mild, moderate, severe or unspecified	Depressive disorders: major depression, dysthymia, unspecified
Bipolar affective disorder	Bipolar disorders: Bipolar I & II, cyclothymia, unspecified
Recurrent depressive disorders	Mood disorder due to a general medical condition
Persistent mood states (dysthymia)	Substance-induced mood disorder
Other mood disorders	Mood disorder not otherwise specified

Table 2.1
Classifications of mood disorders.

Classification

The classification of depressive disorders is important as it helps clinicians to communicate accurately, make uniform diagnoses and plan treatment. An ideal category is one which has distinct clinical features and is well defined in terms of aetiology, response to treatment and outcome. However, few categories fulfil such criteria and there is still much controversy about the definition or even the existence of some subtypes of depression. The reason for this is that the symptoms of depression exist on a continuum. Defining depression involves delineating it from normality and distinguishing it from other psychiatric syndromes. Depressive syndromes have to be defined in terms of severity and duration along a spectrum ranging from normal to pathological mood states. This raises questions about the quality of depression and how to separate this from feelings of unhappiness. Depression is much more than 'feeling low' and, contrary to public perception, it does not involve a weakness of character.[1, 2]

Depressive symptoms can be grouped in a variety of ways, according to their number, severity, frequency, duration and pattern of occurrence. Attempts have also been made to define depressive syndromes by relating them to cause, response to treatment and outcome. With these points in mind the various types of depressive syndrome are described.

ICD-10	DSM-IV
Main symptoms (3)	**Main symptoms (2)**
Depressed mood	Depressed mood
Anhedonia	Anhedonia
Loss of energy	
Additional symptoms	**Additional symptoms**
Altered sleep	Altered sleep
Change of appetite and weight	Change of appetite and weight
Ideas of self-harm or suicide	Ideas of self-harm or suicide
Reduced self-esteem	Fatigue or loss of energy
Feelings of guilt	Feelings of guilt or worthlessness
Reduced concentration	Reduced concentration
Agitation or retardation	Psychomotor agitation or retardation
Impaired functioning	**Impaired functioning**
Duration of symptoms	**Duration of symptoms**
Minimum two-week period with almost daily symptoms	Minimum two-week period with almost daily symptoms

Table 2.2
Symptoms of depression adapted from ICD-10[3] and DSM-IV.[4]

	Main symptoms	Total symptoms (main and additional)
ICD-10		
Mild	2	4
Moderate	2	6
Severe	3	8
DSM-IV	1	5

Table 2.3
Diagnostic criteria for depressive episode (ICD-10 and DSM-IV).

Endogenous and reactive depression

Depression can be categorized as either 'endogenous' or 'exogenous' (more commonly known as reactive or neurotic depression) depending upon the source of causative factors and the symptoms manifested. Endogenous depression, thought to be caused by internal factors, produces biological symptoms of depression, whereas reactive or neurotic depression, thought to be precipitated by external events or stressors, leads to a depressive state with responsive mood and few or no biological symptoms. However, due to heterogeneity within both groups, studies attempting to define endogenous and reactive depression have yielded conflicting findings with only weak supportive evidence in favour of the endogenous–exogenous dichotomy.[5] In practice many patients have a mixture of endogenous and neurotic symptoms so that distinction between the two subtypes can be difficult. Clinicians nevertheless continue to favour the use of these terms, especially endogenous depression because the symptoms help to decide on treatment.

It is important to note that the term neurotic is also used to describe chronic or recurrent minor depression conveying implications of lesser severity and chronicity. Therefore, neurotic depression is a minor depressive state that may persist, and the onset of which is likely to have been related to life events.[6]

Major depression

Defined in both ICD-10 and DSM-IV, major depression sets the standard and consists of affective, behavioural and cognitive components. In major depression, depressed mood is characterized by feelings of guilt and helplessness. Emotional, intellectual and physical functions are often retarded and as a result the patient's verbal and non-verbal communication are diminished, rendering a sense of detachment. The future holds no promise and thoughts focus on past failures and present inadequacy, evoking ideas of hopelessness. Low self-esteem and a feeling of despair prompt ideas of suicide.

Certain symptoms may dominate the clinical presentation, as in agitated depression, where anxiety, manifest as restlessness, is a prominent feature. It is also a relatively common symptom in major depression, although not as prevalent as in minor depressive states. Obsessional and hypochondriacal symptoms also occur frequently, occasionally to the extent of disguising the symptoms of depression.

Psychotic depression

In Britain the term psychotic has been used to describe endogenous depression, differentiating it from neurotic depression. In North America psychotic depression has been used to describe the small number of patients with major depression who develop psychotic symptoms. Delusions of guilt and self-blame preoccupy the patient. Hypochondriacal and nihilistic delusions, concerning body odour, infestation or the rotting of internal organs, dominate the clinical presentation and constantly worry the patient. Motor retardation, if severe, can result in depressive stupor leading to inanition and absent self-care. There is often marked weight loss due to refusal of food and the patient runs the risk of physical ill-health. Suicidal thoughts are often present and should prompt appropriate concern and inquiry.[7]

Minor depression

Minor depression was introduced as part of the Research Diagnostic Criteria (RDC) used by Spitzer[8] at the National Institute of Mental Health (NIMH) to study depression. Although the symptoms used to characterize minor depression are the same as those used to describe major depression, clinically, minor depression is less well defined as its presentation is complicated by somatization and the concurrence of anxiety. Since by definition minor depression is less severe, the symptoms of depression, namely, depressed mood, anhedonia, reduced energy and so on, are less pronounced, making qualitative and quantitative distinctions from normality and anxiety states harder to accomplish.

However, there are certain characteristics of minor depression which can be used for its identification. Minor depression is more likely to result in middle or late insomnia as opposed to initial insomnia which is more characteristic of anxiety states.[9] Similarly, reduced appetite and social functioning are more closely associated with minor depression than with anxiety.[10]

The extensive overlap and admixture of depressive and anxiety symptoms due to the coexistence of two syndromes or the development of one secondary to the other have produced the category of 'mixed anxiety and depression', which given its prevalence may be the usual presentation of these symptoms. In this context, the presence of anxiety symptoms worsens the prognosis.[11]

Dysthymia and double depression

Dysthymia is defined as a chronic depression, usually with an insidious onset, lasting at least two years. A diagnosis of minor or major depression cannot be made because the depressive symptoms are insufficient either in terms of their severity or their duration. Some symptoms, such as guilt and diminished interest, are the same as those found in major depression; however, extremes of retardation or agitation and changes in appetite and weight are less likely.[12] The depression in dysthymia is more subjective than objective, with symptoms of low self-esteem and pessimism being more common, and so distinction from normality is often very difficult. Dysthymia often precedes major depressive episodes and may in some instances continue for the duration of the episode and then persist after it has resolved. Major depression superimposed upon dysthymia is sometimes described as 'double depression'.[13]

Recurrent brief depression

Depressive episodes in recurrent brief depression manifest the same depressive symptoms as major or minor depression. The symptoms recur regularly (at least once a month) over a period of at least one year and usually last less than two weeks but more than two days. It is an important category as response to treatment is particularly poor.[14, 15]

It is important to remember that the symptoms used to define major depression, recurrent brief depression and dysthymia are very similar and that the illnesses overlap considerably. The occurrence of recurrent brief depression together with episodes of major depression is called combined depression.[16]

Atypical depression

Atypical depression is a contentious term that has been used to describe depression with anxiety or pain as a prominent symptom, depression with reversed biological symptoms and depression without somatic symptoms. It is included as a specifier in DSM-IV and can be applied to both major depression and dysthymia. The classic features of atypical depression are those described by the Columbia group and include hypersomnia and hyperphagia, amongst others (summarized in *Table 2.4*). Monoamine oxidase inhibitors (MAOIs) are thought to be more suited to the treatment of atypical depression than other antidepressants, particularly phenelzine.[17, 18]

Chronic depression

Chronic depression involves a heterogeneous group consisting of depressive states in which the symptoms fail to fulfil criteria for any syndromes.[19] Akiskal[12, 20] has attempted to subdivide chronic depression into various subtypes. However, the definitions are too imprecise and there are no agreed criteria for chronicity. It should be noted that chronicity does not equate with severity or treatment resistance and simply describes the persistence of depressive symptoms. Some chronic depressions are the residual state that follows incomplete recovery from a depressive episode; others are thought to be 'characterological' and are associated with personality problems. Depression secondary to physical illness or that which is treatment resistant is often diagnosed as chronic depression. Therefore at present the term chronic depression is perhaps too vague and should be avoided. Instead the individual symptoms should be described, specifying their duration.

Resistant depression

Treatment-resistant depression is that which persists despite appropriate treatment. The definition of resistant depression is dependent upon correct diagnosis and

Table 2.4
Features of atypical depression.

- Depressed but reactive mood (mood improves in positive milieu)
- Reversed diurnal variation of mood
- Increase in weight and appetite (particularly carbohydrates)
- Increased sleep
- Excessive fatigue
- Interpersonal rejection sensitivity

accurate assessment. Failed treatments should be specified and all alternative aetiologies excluded[21] (this is considered further in *Chapter 8*).[22]

Depression in bipolar affective disorder

Bipolar affective disorder is that in which, in addition to depressive episodes, a patient suffers episodes of elevated mood (mania, hypomania). It seems to have a distinct biological basis biochemically and genetically, starting earlier in life than unipolar depression and affecting men and women in equal numbers. Following a manic episode the management of bipolar affective disorder involves the use of anti-manic and mood-stabilizing drugs, and the treatment of further depressive episodes with antidepressant medication risks precipitating mania. The management of bipolar affective disorders is therefore very different and is not discussed.[23]

Epidemiology

Depression is associated with widespread and significant functional disability. It is a recurrent, often chronic, illness with serious and far-reaching consequences.

Depressive disorders are under-recognized and even when detected and correctly diagnosed they are often inappropriately managed. The epidemiology of depressive disorders has highlighted these problems and provides a valuable means of surveying depressive disorders and monitoring their treatment. Epidemiological data are particularly useful when attempting to predict the course of an illness, its likely response to treatment and eventual outcome.

Major depression is a common illness. It affects approximately 3% of the general population at any one time (point prevalence). Over a period of a year this figure doubles to about 6% and the lifetime prevalence is three times this — that is, 16–18%. Women experience depression more often than men, with a lifetime incidence of 1 in 5 as compared with 1 in 10 for men. The average age for onset of major depression is about 40 years and, in 50% of cases, depression first occurs between the ages of 20 and 50 years. The peak age of onset of major depression is in the mid-20s although it can occur at any age from childhood onwards. It is interesting to note that the age of onset has become progressively younger, suggesting perhaps an increasing susceptibility to the illness or increased awareness.[24, 25]

The prevalence of dysthymia, at any one time or over a time period, is approximately the same, at around 3%. However, it is of note that many patients with dysthymia suffer episodes of major depression which may go undetected or are recorded as major depressive disorder instead of 'double depression'.[26] Similarly the prevalence of recurrent brief depression differs in various studies due to differences in diagnosis and patient characteristics. The reported prevalence of recurrent brief depression over a period of a year is between 5 and 7% and the lifetime prevalence is between 10 and 15%.[27]

The point prevalence of depressive symptoms is approximately 20% and over a period of one year this increases the risk of developing major depression four-fold.[28] Minor depression has a one year and point prevalence of about 2% but its lifetime prevalence is much higher at around 10%.

It is important to note that the various diagnoses can change over time and in many cases there are comorbid psychiatric illnesses which affect the course and outcome of the depressive disorder.[29]

Overall recent studies using modern methodology have yielded higher prevalence rates of most mood disorders *(Table 2.5)*.

Depressive disorder	Prevalence — one year (%)	Prevalence — lifetime (%)
Minor depression	2	10
Dysthymia	3	3
Brief recurrent depression	6	12
Major depression	6	17

Table 2.5
Prevalence rates for mood disorders (approximate).

Key Points

- Clinically, the diagnosis of depressive disorders is best made by eliciting the characteristic signs and symptoms of depression.

- The specific clinical features of depression, its duration, severity and response to treatment, determine its particular sub-type.

- There are many 'sub-types' of depression:
  minor and major depression
  psychotic depression
  endogenous depression (melancholia)
  reactive (neurotic) depression
  atypical depression
  agitated depression
  dysthymia and double depression
  recurrent brief depression and combined depression
  chronic depression
  treatment-resistant depression
  mixed anxiety and depression
  some have pharmacological specificity.

- Depressive disorders are common, occurring at all ages, in both sexes and often in conjunction with other illnesses.

References

1.   Winokar G. All roads lead to depression: clinically homogenous, aetiologically heterogenous. *Journal of Affective Disorders* (1997) 45: 97–108.

2.   Kendler KS, Gardner CO. Boundaries of major depression: an evaluation of DSM-IV criteria. *American Journal of Psychiatry* (1998) 155: 172–7.

3. World Health Organization. *ICD-10 Classification of Mental and Behavioural Disorders. Clinical Descriptions and Diagnostic Guidelines* (Geneva: WHO, 1992).

4. American Psychiatric Association. *Diagnostic and Statistical Manual of Mental Disorders*, 4th edn (Washington, DC: American Psychiatric Association, 1994).

5. Kendall RE. The classification of depressions: a review of contemporary confusion. *British Journal of Psychiatry* (1976) **129**: 15–28.

6. Grove WM, Andreasen NC. Concepts, diagnosis and classification. In: Paykel ES ed, *Handbook of Affective Disorders*, 2nd edn (London: Churchill Livingstone, 1992) 25–41.

7. Coryell W. The treatment of psychotic depression. *Journal of Clinical Psychiatry* (1998) **59 (suppl 1)**: 22–7.

8. Spitzer R, Endicott J, Robins E. Research diagnostic criteria: rationale and reliability. *Archives of General Psychiatry* (1978) **35**: 773–82.

9. Kupfer DJ, Thase ME. Laboratory studies and validity of psychiatric diagnosis: has there been any progress? In: Robins LN, Barret JE eds, *The Validity of Psychiatric Diagnosis* (New York: Raven Press, 1989) 177–202.

10. Angst J. Depression and anxiety: a review of studies in the community and in primary health care. In: Sartorius N, Goldgerg D, de Girolamo G et al eds, *Psychological Disorders in General Medical Settings* (Toronto: Hogrefe & Huber, 1990) 60–8.

11. Nutt D. Management of patients with depression associated with anxiety symptoms. *Journal of Clinical Psychiatry* (1997) **58 (suppl 8)**: 11–16.

12. Akiskal HS. Dysthymic disorder: psychopathology of proposed chronic depressive subtypes. *American Journal of Psychiatry* (1983) **140**: 11–20.

13. Keller MB, Shapiro RW. 'Double Depression' superimposition of acute depressive episodes on chronic depressive disorders. *American Journal of Psychiatry* (1982) **139**: 438–42.

14. Angst J. The history and concept of recurrent brief depression. *European Archives of Psychiatry and Clinical Neuroscience* (1994) **244**: 171–3.

15. Montgomery DB, Roberts A, Green M et al. Lack of efficacy of fluoxetine in recurrent brief depression and suicidal attempts. *European Archives of Psychiatry and Clinical Neuroscience* (1994) **244**: 211–15.

16. Angst J. Dysthymia and the spectrum of chronic depressions. In: Akiskal HS, Cassano GB eds, *Minor and Recurrent Brief Depression* (New York, London: Guildford Press, 1997) 183–90.

17. Liebowitz MR, Quitkin FM, Stewart JW et al. Antidepressant specificity in atypical depression. *Archives of General Psychiatry* (1988) **45**: 129–37.

18. Quitkin FM, Stewart JW, McGrath PJ. Columbia atypical depression. *British Journal of Psychiatry* (1993) **163 (suppl)**: 30–4.

19. Scott J. Chronic depression. *British Journal of Psychiatry* (1988) **153**: 287–97.

20. Akiskal HS. Validating affective personality types. In: Robins LN ed, *The Validity of Psychiatric Diagnoses* (New York: Raven Press, 1989) 217–27.

21. Bridges PK, Hodgkiss AD, Malizia AL. Practical management of treatment-resistant affective disorders. *British Journal of Hospital Medicine* (1995) **54**: 501–6.

22. Bowskill RJ, Bridges PK. Treatment-resistant affective disorders. *British Journal of Hospital Medicine* (1997) 57: 171–2.

23. Montgomery SA, Cassano GB. *Management of Bipolar Disorder* (London: Martin Dunitz, 1996).

24. Weissmann MM, Bland RC, Canino GJ. Cross-national epidemiology of major depression and bipolar disorder. *Journal of the American Medical Association* (1996) **276**: 293–9.

25. Kessler RC, McGonagle KA, Zhao S. Lifetime and 12-month prevalence of DSM-III-R psychiatric disorders in the United States: results of the National Comorbidity Survey. *Archives of General Psychiatry* (1994) **51**: 8–19.

26. Angst J. The epidemiology of dysthymia. In: Fahy TA, Joughin NA, Kent A et al eds, *Psychiatry: Peer Selected Citations* (London: Current Medical Literature, 1996) 6–11.

27. Angst J, Merikangas KR, Preisig M. Subthreshold syndromes of depression and anxiety in the community. *Journal of Clinical Psychiatry* (1997) **58 (suppl 18)**: 6–10.

28. Howarth E, Johnson J, Klerman GL et al. Depressive symptoms as relative and attributable risk factors for first-onset major depression. *Archives of General Psychiatry* (1992) **49**: 817–23.

29. Lepine J, Gastpar M, Mendlewicz J et al. Depression in the community: the first pan-European study DEPRES (Depression Research in European Society). *International Clinical Psychopharmacology* (1997) **12**: 19–29.

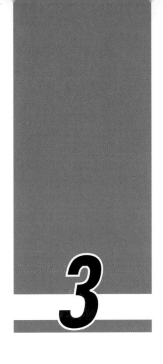

Assessment and investigation of depression

Introduction

The clinical evaluation of a depressed patient varies according to the setting of the consultation, depending upon the resources available and the personalities of both patient and clinician. It consists of a systematic assessment and relevant investigations. In this chapter the various components of these are discussed in turn. Occasionally investigations are carried out for the purposes of research and these are considered separately at the end.

Presentation

Upon first contact it is important to establish how the patient has presented, tracing previous contacts and collating as much information as possible from referrers, informants and collateral sources such as previous notes. This is particularly important with severe illnesses where the patient may not be able to provide sufficient or indeed accurate information.

Patients presenting to their GP may be referred to a psychiatrist for specialist help, who in turn may sometimes seek a further opinion. On each occasion the diagnosis should be confirmed, even when the patient is well known and has a long-standing history of depressive illness. The possibility of an underlying physical illness and a comorbid or even another psychiatric disorder should be considered.

Upon presentation the priorities are to establish or reaffirm the diagnosis, to explore the possibility of other concurrent illnesses, and to ascertain how the patient has presented and why at this time. The last point is important in terms of understanding the depressive illness and its possible causes.

History

The psychiatric history of a depressed patient should address the points in *Table 3.1*. Some of these are discussed further.

Informants

The presenting symptoms of depression have been described in *Chapter 1*, and the grouping of these to help formulate a

---

- **Family history** — specifically of an affective disorder, alcoholism, physical disorders
- **Pre-morbid personality** — involvement of informants is essential for accurate appraisal
- **Past psychiatric history** — depression, substance abuse, anxiety disorders, eating disorders and psychosis
- **Social history** — current living conditions, employment, partner, dependants, finances and habits/hobbies
- **Medical and pharmacotherapeutic history** — illnesses and medications that can cause depression
- **Psychiatric therapies** — psychological and pharmacological, noting suitability of treatments and response
- **Suicidality** — past history of any self-harm, current suicidal intent

Table 3.1
Key points in the psychiatric history of a depressed patient.

diagnosis has been discussed in **Chapter 2**. A careful record of these and the patient's mental state is important for subsequent management. Observations concerning the course of an illness and its response to treatment depend upon the quality of the information gathered. It is therefore necessary that the patient's subjective account of psychological symptoms be corroborated from as many collateral sources as possible as unusual behaviour may only be revealed in this way. This usually involves consultation with family members or friends. The nature of any prior contact with medical services should also be explored, particularly if it has involved psychiatric intervention. Copies of the original notes or at least the relevant summaries can often be obtained and, in complicated cases, it may be necessary to talk directly to the healthcare professionals previously involved.

Family history

The genetics of depression, discussed in **Chapter 4**, naturally influence its course and prognosis. However, a family history of depression is also important because it will have a bearing on what support the family can provide. A patient with a family history of depression probably has a better understanding of the illness but is also likely to have different expectations as concerns management. Within a family the presence of an additional member with a psychiatric illness may prove to be too grave a burden. The social consequences of depression need careful evaluation and the patient and family members may need additional support. It is not uncommon for marriages to break up and the patient to be blamed for the failings of other individuals. A supportive family member is a great asset and should be involved in the management of the patient as far as possible.

Psychiatric history

The onset of depression is often difficult to specify, particularly as there is often an insidious emergence of psychological symptoms. Symptoms of depression can be masked by the presence of physical problems and, if set against a background of social adversity, the patient may not acknowledge their existence, perceiving them instead as an understandable corollary. The treatments received and the clinical response to them can also be difficult to assess, especially if the history obtained is complicated, extensive or incomplete. In such cases the use of a life chart may be helpful. In this the patient's mood, treatments and significant life events are plotted against time. A lot of information can be summarized in this manner, and an example is given in *Figure 3.1*.

Treatment history

When reviewing the history of depression it is important to note the treatments that have been prescribed at every stage of the

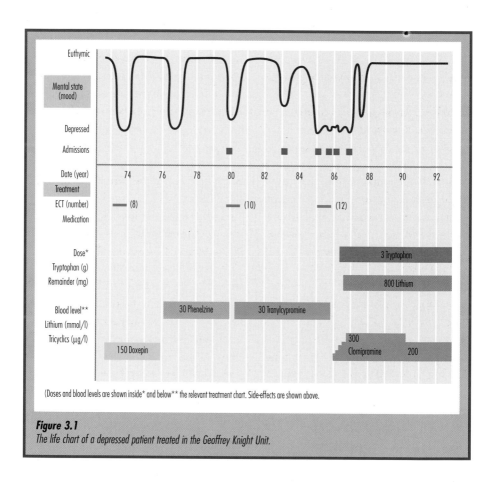

(Doses and blood levels are shown inside* and below** the relevant treatment chart. Side-effects are shown above.

Figure 3.1
The life chart of a depressed patient treated in the Geoffrey Knight Unit.

illness. The adequacy of any treatment, its suitability and efficacy, needs to be assessed. Naturally this applies to both psychological and physical treatments, but here we shall focus on the evaluation of pharmacological interventions, as this is frequently carried out inadequately. The aspects of pharmacotherapy that need to be noted are discussed in turn.

Dose, compliance and therapeutic drug monitoring

The dose of any antidepressant used in the treatment of depressive illness should be sufficient to attain a therapeutic blood level. In most cases knowledge of the dose alone is of little practical value because the antidepressant blood levels of patients on the same dose of medication can be very different. For many antidepressants the relationship between dose and blood level is complex because individuals' metabolic characteristics vary.[1] A 'therapeutic range', specifying upper and lower limits, has been suggested for only a few antidepressants[2,3] and, in practice, it is evident that low levels of antidepressants are likely to be ineffective whilst high levels can cause side-effects.

The concept of a therapeutic range is less useful when applied to some of the newer antidepressants such as the selective serotonin reuptake inhibitors (SSRIs), as there is little correlation between blood levels

and clinical response.[4,5] Nevertheless, measuring the blood levels is a useful means of assessing compliance and preventing any possible toxicity.

In routine clinical practice the antidepressant dosages used are often inadequate.[6] This is particularly the case in general practice where, because of the possibility of side effects, low doses of tricyclics are often prescribed.[7] This is less of a problem with the newer antidepressants as they are usually prescribed at a fixed dose.[8]

The pharmacokinetic and pharmacodynamic interactions of antidepressants can result in the elevation of their blood levels or an increase in their breakdown and metabolism and so the monitoring of antidepressant blood levels is useful when combining drugs. The side-effects of antidepressants affect compliance and so, clinically, the dose of an antidepressant should be titrated upwards, balancing side-effects against therapeutic benefit. However, in this scenario it is important to remember that the delay in clinical response is likely to favour non-compliance, especially if the side-effects are not anticipated or are particularly troublesome. Warning the patient about side-effects and the delay in efficacy is likely to encourage compliance and imbue confidence in the treatment strategy.[9]

Treatment response and patterns of treatment

The delay in onset of action of antidepressants is well recognized but poorly understood. Tricyclic antidepressants and SSRIs take effect after 2–6 weeks of treatment at a therapeutic dose, whereas MAOIs take almost twice as long.[10] Many claim that certain treatment strategies have a faster onset of action. However, none have been convincingly substantiated. It is worth while noting that depression can spontaneously remit and that an apparent response to treatment may be because of this or due to a placebo effect. Nevertheless many types of depression benefit from antidepressant treatment and the response is relatively even and predictable in comparison with other reasons for improvement.[11, 12] The likelihood of response seems to depend upon the type of depression. Endogenous features predict a good response to antidepressants and improvement early in treatment suggests ultimately a more positive response.

The stages of antidepressant treatment and patterns of response are shown in *Figure 3.2*. In practice, it is important to be familiar with the various stages of treatment and to be able to differentiate between the relapse and recurrence of depressive symptoms. Clinical improvement has three phases: response to treatment, remission of symptoms and complete recovery.

A reduction in the severity or number of symptoms is described as a *response*. The eventual absence of symptoms is described as *remission*, and the return of normal mood and social functioning is described as *recovery*. Prior to complete recovery the recrudescence of symptoms is described as a *relapse*, whereas following recovery it is described as a *recurrence. Acute treatment* stabilizes the presenting symptoms leading to remission. *Continuation treatment* aims to prevent a relapse of the illness and to lead to recovery. *Maintenance treatment* is continued beyond recovery and attempts to prevent a recurrence of the illness.

Treatment duration

Following an episode of major depression more than 50% of patients will have another in their lifetime, and of these 80–90% are likely to suffer yet further episodes.[13, 14] In the majority of cases (75–80%), major depression is a recurrent illness. However, 20% only ever suffer one episode of depression. With each new

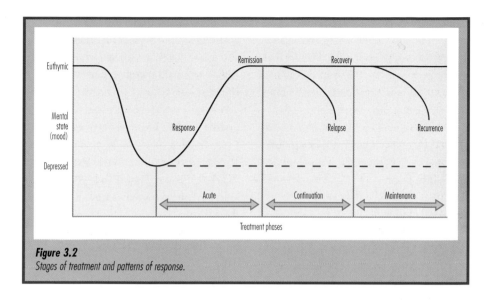

Figure 3.2
Stages of treatment and patterns of response.

depressive episode, the period between episodes decreases and the illness increases both in severity and resistance to treatment so that, eventually, a fifth of patients develop chronic depression.[15] Consequently there is a need for continuation and maintenance treatment aimed at attaining recovery and preventing recurrence. It is important to note that medication used in the acute phase of treatment is likely to be continued during maintenance treatment and that compliance can only be sustained if it is tolerated by the patient when recovered. Hence the initial choice of antidepressant has long-term implications and these need to be considered when deciding upon treatment.

The appropriate duration of treatment is a clinical decision. The presence of residual symptoms increases the likelihood of relapse and so treatment should continue until the patient is symptom-free. Even after this stage, ideally, treatment should continue for a further 4–5 months.[16] If after this period of time depressive symptoms re-emerge then this can be considered a recurrence, as opposed to a relapse, and be dealt with as has been discussed. It is important to note that the premature withdrawal of medication may encourage relapse, and so the discontinuation of treatment should be a timely planned event and not one that is initiated by the patient because of intolerable side-effects.

Table 3.2 shows some of the steps involved in a typical evaluation of a severely depressed patient, outlining the members of a psychiatric team who may be involved.

Investigations

Investigations are usually carried out as part of the initial assessment of a depressed patient. They may also be indicated when there is a change in the mental or physical health of the patient or the treatment is modified. The routine investigations are briefly discussed and summarised in *Table 3.3*.

Routine investigations

A full blood count, including haemoglobin and red blood cell parameters, may reveal anaemia, B12 and folate deficiencies. Chronically depressed patients may develop these problems by having neglected their diet. Anaemia due to blood loss or iron deficiency often presents as fatigue. B12 and folate deficiencies can compromise cognitive function and produce confusional states. Infections can also cause depression and these may be detected by finding a raised white cell count.

Metabolic function can be investigated by checking urea and electrolyte plasma levels. Disturbances may arise due to dehydration or physical illness and are important to note, not only to detect underlying pathology but also to ensure that treatments can be prescribed safely. For instance, lithium should not be prescribed in conditions of sodium imbalance, and all types of antidepressants can cause hyponatraemia due to the inappropriate secretion of antidiuretic hormone.

Abnormalities of the thyroid often lead to depression and so thyroid function tests should be performed routinely, particularly upon initial investigation. Liver function tests are important as they can reveal alcohol abuse; however, very many antidepressants alter liver function and so this needs to be taken into consideration.

Additional investigations

Most of these are conducted in hospital. The investigations and indications are summarised in *Table 3.4*.

- **Psychiatric history** — from patient, informants, past records; see *Table 3.1*
- **Haematological and biochemical investigations** — see *Table 3.4*
- **Social assessments** — e.g. living conditions, involving social workers and community team members
- **Psychological assessments** — to detect specific problems or assess suitability for therapy
- **Nursing and occupational therapist assessments** — to evaluate level of functioning

Table 3.2
Aspects of psychiatric assessment.

- Full blood count (haemoglobin, white blood cell count, red blood cell indices)
- B12 and folate
- Urea and electrolytes (plasma sodium and potassium concentration)
- Plasma calcium
- Thyroid function tests
- Liver function tests

Table 3.3
Routine biochemical and haematological investigations.

Investigation	Indications
Antidepressant blood levels	To ensure compliance or avoid toxicity
Urinary drug screen	To confirm suspected drug abuse, eg cannabis use
Electrocardiogram (ECG)	Prior to ECT and sometimes with high-dose antidepressants
Computed tomography (brain)	If intracranial pathology is suspected

Table 3.4
Additional investigations.

Research investigations

Some investigations are carried out for the
purposes of research and these are shown
in *Table 3.5*.

- Electroencephalography (EEG)
- Structural and functional neuroimaging
- Sleep studies
- Hormone tests (dexamethazone suppression test, neuroendocrine challenge tests)
- Metabolic investigations of precursors and metabolites in urine, blood and cerebrospinal fluid (CSF)

Table 3.5
Research investigations.[17]

Key Points

- The key points in the psychiatric history of a depressed patient *(Table 3.1)* should be corroborated from as many reliable sources as possible, for example previous medical notes, relatives and friends.

- It is especially important to critically reappraise all the treatments that the patient has received. With respect to medication it is necessary to check that compliance has been adequately ensured and that suitable doses of appropriate antidepressants have been used for sufficient duration.

- The necessary investigations *(Tables 3.3* and *3.4)* should be conducted to exclude any physical causes of depression.

- The successful assessment and investigation of a depressed patient requires a **multidisciplinary approach**, for instance:

  - **doctors** — elicit psychiatric symptoms and carry out investigations

  - **nurses** — perform clinical assessments and maintain the necessary observation and support of patients (at home and in hospitals)

  - **psychologists** — conduct psychological evaluation

  - **social workers** — appraise social needs and functioning

  - **occupational therapists** — determine work and daily living capabilities.

References

1. Preskorn SH. Pharmacokinetics of antidepressants: why and how they are relevant to treatment. *Journal Of Clinical Psychiatry* (1993) **54 (suppl 14-34)**: 55–6.

2. Breyer-Pfaff U, Giedke H, Gaertner HJ et al. Validation of a therapeutic plasma level range in amitriptyline treatment of depression. *Journal of Clinical Psychopharmacology* (1989) 9: 116–21.

3. Balant-Gorgia AE, Gex-Fabry M, Balant LP. Clinical pharmacokinetics of clomipramine. *Clinical Pharmacokinetics* (1991) **20**: 447–62.

4. Bauman P, Rochat B. Comparative pharmacokinetics of selective serotonin reuptake inhibitors: a look behind the mirror. *International Clinical Psychopharmacology* (1995) **10 (suppl 1)**: 15–21.

5. Glassman AH. Antidepressant plasma levels revisited. Symposium on Management of Treatment-Resistant Depression (1993, Rio de Janerio, Brazil). *International Clinical Psychopharmacology* (1994) **9 (suppl 2)**: 25–30.

6. Bridges PK. '...and a small dose of antidepressant might help'. *British Journal of Psychiatry* (1983) **142**: 626–8.

7. Munizza C, Tibaldi G, Bollini E et al. Prescription pattern of antidepressants in out-patient psychiatric practice. *Psychological Medicine* (1995) **25**: 771–8.

8. Donoghue JM. A comparison of prescribing patterns of selective serotonin reuptake inhibitors in the treatment of depression in primary care in the United Kingdom. *Journal of Serotonin Research* (1995) **1**: 47–51.

9. Fernando MLD, Kazarian SS. Patient education in the drug treatment of psychiatric disorders. *CNS Drugs* (1995) **3**: 291–304.

10. Danjou P, Weiller E, Richardot P. Onset of action of antidepressants: a literature survey. In: Langer SZ, Brunello N, Racagni G et al. eds, *Critical Issues in the Treatment of Affective Disorders* (Basel: Karger, 1994) 136–53.

11. Paykel ES, Hollyman JA, Freeling P et al. Predictors of therapeutic benefit from amitriptyline in mild depression: a general practice placebo-controlled trial. *Journal of Affective Disorders* (1988) **14**: 83–95.

12. Quitkin FM, Rabkin JG, Ross D et al. Identification of true drug response to antidepressants. *Archives of General Psychiatry* (1984) **41**: 782–6.

13. Kupfer DJ. Long-term management of depression. *Journal Of Clinical Psychiatry* (1991) **52 (suppl 5):** 28–34.

14. Angst J. How recurrent and predictable is depressive illness? In: Montgomery S, Rouillon F eds, *Perspectives in Psychiatry* (Chichester: Wiley, 1992) 1–13.

15. Thase ME. Long-term treatments of recurrent depressive disorders. *Journal of Clinical Psychiatry* (1992) **53 (suppl 9)**: 32–44.

16. Prien RF, Kupfer DJ. Continuation drug therapy for major depressive episodes: how long should it be maintained? *American Journal of Psychiatry* (1986) **143**: 18–23.

17. Trimble MR. Affective disorders. In: *Biological Psychiatry* 2nd Edition.(Chichester: Wiley, 1996) 226–65.

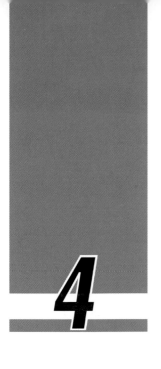

Biological basis of depression

Brain biology and biochemistry are central to the multi-factorial aetiology of depression. Here we examine the biological basis of depression and how it responds to treatment.

A biological view of the causes of depression begins with the study of genes. These provide the organism with its physiological essence, from which, by means of growth and development, its defining characteristics and attributes are attained. Influences, both within the organism and between it and its environment, are mediated by biochemical means. Thus the biological aetiology of depression can be considered from genetic and biochemical perspectives.

Genetics of depression

The degree to which genes contribute to depressive illness has traditionally been investigated using family, twin and adoption studies. Important in this has been the need to determine whether depression is familial because of a shared environment or the possession of common genetic material. The aggregation of depressive illnesses in families has revealed that both unipolar and bipolar depression breed true and that the risk to an individual, from the same family as someone who is already affected, is approximately doubled. Research comparing the concordance rates of monozygotic and dizygotic twins has shown that, although the heritability of depression is greater for bipolar illness, it is also a factor in unipolar illness and probably plays a significant role in its causation.[1-4] These findings from family and twin studies are further supported by studies examining the contrasting rates of illness between biological and adoptive parents of affected individuals, which show that the natural parents of affected adoptees have greater rates of depression.[5-7]

Genetic marker studies have used association studies and techniques such as linkage analysis to study the genetics of mood disorders. Results from such research examining the association of genetic markers with disease genes are promising, particularly concerning bipolar illness in which the findings indicate that a single gene of significant effect is unlikely and that several genes are probably involved. Significant proportions of those with familial bipolar illness have links to loci on specific chromosomes; however, ultimately, it seems that the development of depressive disorders involves a number of genes, each of small effect and varying influence.[8]

The environmental causes of depression are thought to contribute to the variations in onset and expression of the illness seen in clinical practice. One of the main links between environmental influences and biological changes in depression is thought to be the stress (hypothalamic–pituitary–adrenal — HPA) axis which, when activated, leads to the release of hormones such as cortisol (see later in this chapter). Cortisol can itself cause symptoms of depression and, indeed, its secretion is associated with many aspects of the illness, including its environmental causative factors. For instance, severe life events increase the release of cortisol in depressives whereas social support is thought to diminish this.[9, 10]

It is noteworthy that neither genes nor the environment are wholly responsible for causing depression and that this is also true when considering the biochemical aspects of depression.

Biochemistry of depression

The biochemical aspects of depression can be considered under the headings of neurochemistry and neuroendocrinology.

Neurochemistry of depression

At about the same time as when antidepressants were discovered, it was noted that reserpine, an antihypertensive agent, when administered to some patients, caused symptoms of depression. Studies revealed that reserpine depleted neuronal monoamine neurotransmitters, noradrenaline (NA), dopamine (DA) and serotonin (5-HT), and that this was probably responsible for its depressant action. Conversely, tricyclic antidepressants and monoamine oxidase inhibitors enhanced monoamine neurotransmission by increasing the availability of neurotransmitters in the synapse. Imipramine was found to do this by inhibiting presynaptic neuronal reuptake of noradrenaline and serotonin, while the monoamine oxidase inhibitors achieved the same by inhibiting the degradation of neurotransmitter monoamines. It was these observations that led to the monoamine theory of depression. The theory suggested that depression was a consequence of diminished monoaminergic neurotransmission due to a decrease in monoamines, or a reduction of receptor sensitivity at specific monoaminergic receptor sites.[11, 12]

However, the biochemical changes found in depression have not been explained by a single model or theory, and it is now thought probable that many neurotransmitter systems, acting at various sites within the brain, participate with neuroendocrine mechanisms in the pathogenesis of depressive illness.[13]

To understand the actions of antidepressants it is necessary to be familiar with the process of neurotransmission. This is, therefore, briefly described in general terms, and the specifics of individual systems are summarised in their respective diagrams and tables.

Neuronal neurotransmission

Chemical neurotransmission is one of the methods by which neurones transfer or exchange information *(Figure 4.1)*. It takes place at chemical synapses which consist of a specific region where the membranes of two neurones are in close proximity. Neurotransmitters are chemicals that carry the information between neurones, and they exert their effects at specific pre- or post-synaptic receptors.

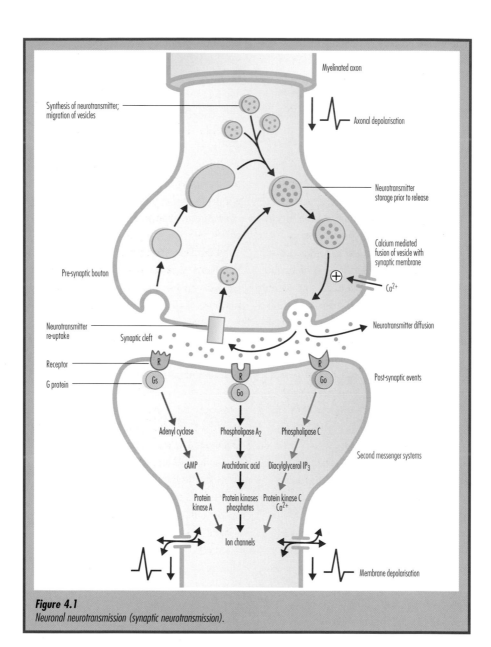

Figure 4.1
Neuronal neurotransmission (synaptic neurotransmission).

The whole process takes only a few milliseconds and is the culmination of many steps.[14]

The neurotransmitter is usually synthesized within the neurone and then transported and stored, prior to its release, at the pre-synaptic membrane. Release of the neurotransmitter into the synaptic cleft is triggered by calcium-dependent depolarization, and the process is often modulated by autoreceptor function. Once within the synaptic cleft, the neurotransmitter binds to its specific receptors and its action is then terminated by diffusion, metabolism or reuptake into the pre-synaptic neurone. The specific receptor binding of a neurotransmitter leads to a series of events, collectively known as transduction, and, following this, the neurone bearing the receptor develops a biological response.[14]

The metabolism and receptor interactions of the monoamine neurotransmitters, NA and 5-HT, are summarized in *Figures 4.2–4.6* and *Tables 4.1* and *4.2*. The pharmacological actions of some of the antidepressants are also illustrated.

Neuroendocrinology of depression

Essential aspects of the HPA axis are summarized in *Figure 4.7*.

The HPA axis is the core stress axis in humans, which shows activation in response not only to physical stressors such as infection but also to psychological stressors in the form of adverse life events. Activation of the axis is essential for the maintenance of normal physiological homeostasis. The end-organ hormone, cortisol, is essential for human survival. Inability to secrete cortisol in response to a stressor is incompatible with life.

Abnormalities in the HPA have been the most consistently demonstrated biological markers in depressive illness. In more severe forms of depression, patients hypersecrete cortisol and show significant adrenal gland enlargement. Many of these patients also fail to suppress cortisol in response to dexamethasone challenge.[15] The hypothalamic peptide corticotrophin-releasing hormone (CRH) is available as a synthetic peptide and can be given intravenously. Patients with major depression

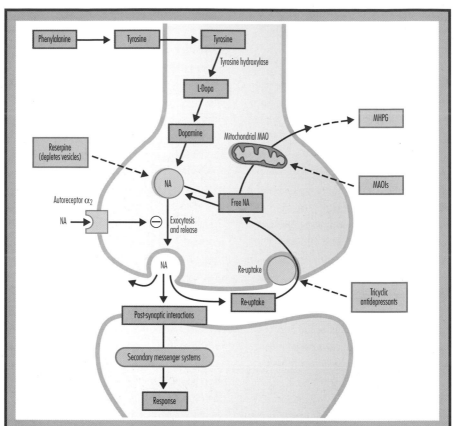

Figure 4.2

L-phenylalanine is the dietary precursor of tyrosine, which is actively taken up by the neurone and then hydroxylated and decarboxylated to form dopamine. This is how dopamine synthesis is achieved in dopaminergic neurones. However, in noradrenergic neurones, the dopamine is hydroxylated to form noradrenaline which is then stored in vesicles awaiting calcium-dependent exocytosis and release. Intrasynaptic noradrenaline acts on pre- and post-synaptic receptors. Its action is terminated by diffusion, breakdown or reuptake. Pre-synaptic neuronal reuptake is inhibited by tricyclic antidepressants. Mitochondrial monoamine oxidase (MAO) metabolizes free intraneuronal noradrenaline and the products of this undergo further degradation and eventual urinary excretion. There are two isoenzymes of MAO. MAO-A is responsible for the metabolism of NA and 5HT, and MAO-B is responsible for the metabolism of tyramine and dopamine. The receptor interactions of NA lead to a cascade of events involving second messenger systems which ultimately produce a physiological response.

MHPG = 3-methoxy-4-hydroxyphenylglycol

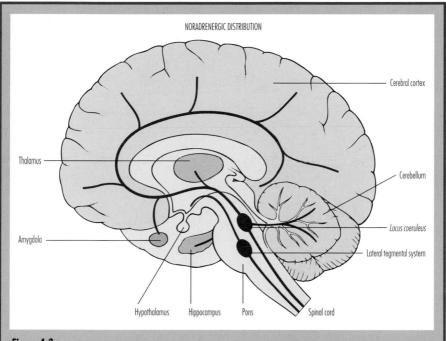

NORADRENERGIC DISTRIBUTION

Cerebral cortex

Thalamus

Cerebellum

Locus coeruleus

Amygdala

Lateral tegmental system

Hypothalamus   Hippocampus   Pons   Spinal cord

Figure 4.3
Noradrenegic neurones are concentrated in the brainstem and hypothalamus. There are two main groups of noradrenergic cell bodies, namely, the locus coeruleus and the lateral tegmental system. The locus coeruleus is situated in the floor of the fourth ventricle of the pons. Noradrenergic neurones innervate the thalamus, hypothalamus, hippocampus, cortex and subcortical limbic regions.

show significant blunting of adrenocorticotrophic hormone (ACTH) release in response to CRH infusion. Studies of cerebrospinal fluid indicate increased levels of CRH in depression.[16] This hypersecretion of CRH is associated with elevated secretion of ACTH. It is clear, therefore, that in depression abnormalities occur at every level of the HPA.[17]

Numerous other neuroendocrine disturbances have also been reported in depression. These include blunted clonidine-induced growth hormone

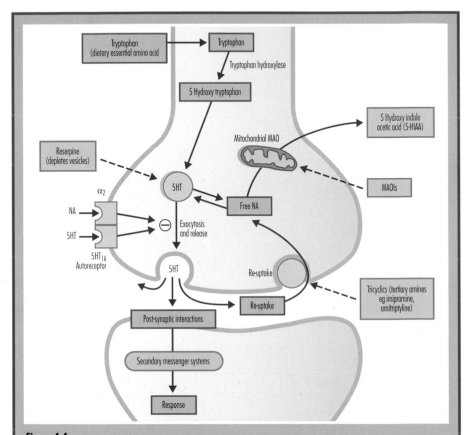

Figure 4.4

Serotonin (5HT) is synthesized from an essential amino acid, tryptophan. Following synthesis it is stored in vesicles prior to its release into the synaptic cleft. Its reuptake is via a specific pre-synaptic transporter which can be inhibited by SSRIs and tertiary tricyclic antidepressants. Like noradrenaline, free intraneuronal 5HT can be metabolized by mitochondrial MAO. Intrasynaptic 5HT acts on post-synaptic receptors producing physiological responses and on pre-synaptic 5HT$_{1A}$ autoreceptors to inhibit further 5HT release. The release of 5HT is also inhibited by noradrenergic neurones via pre-synaptic α-$_2$ heteroreceptors. This inhibitory effect of noradrenaline upon the axons and pre-synaptic terminals of serotonergic neurones is opposite to its excitatory effect on serotonin cell bodies and dendrites, which it achieves via post-synaptic α-$_1$ receptors **(Figure 4.6)**.

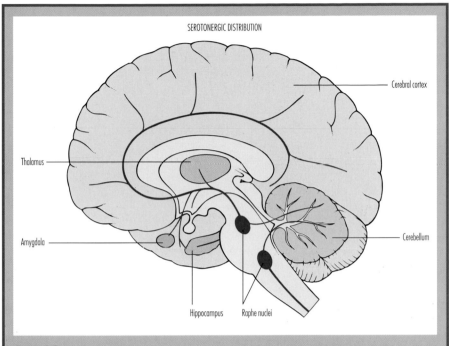

SEROTONERGIC DISTRIBUTION

Cerebral cortex

Thalamus

Amygdala

Cerebellum

Hippocampus   Raphe nuclei

Figure 4.5
Serotonin cell bodies are found in the raphe nuclei, in the pontomedullary region of the brainstem. The nuclei form broadly two groups from which the major ascending tract is the median forebrain bundle. Serotonergic fibres innervate the hippocampus, amygdala, thalamus, hypothalamus, cerebellum and cerbral cortex, and 5HT plays a significant role in aggression, appetite, the sleep—wake cycle and cardio-respiratory homeostasis, in addition to its complex involvement in modifying mood.

release, indicative of central α-2 adreno-ceptor dysfunction. Several research groups have investigated serotonergic-mediated prolactin release. The 5-HT releasing agent and reuptake inhibitor, fenfluramine, has been used in such studies. In patients with major depression a blunted release of prolactin is seen and

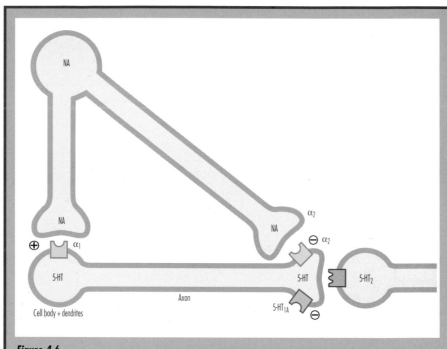

Figure 4.6
The sophisticated interaction of the two main systems modified by antidepressant pharmacotherapy is briefly described. Serotonergic neurotransmission can be facilitated by noradrenergic action via α-1 adrenoceptors. These are post-synaptic receptors on serotonin neuronal cell bodies or dendrites. Stimulation of these adrenoceptors enhances serotonin neurotransmission. Conversely, noradrenergic influence upon serotonergic neurotransmission can be inhibitory, as pre-synaptic α-2 adrenoceptors on serotonergic neurones, when stimulated, inhibit the release of serotonin.

is interpreted as indicating a serotonergic receptor subsensitivity.[18]

It can be argued that chronic stress, which activates the HPA, will in certain susceptible people produce changes in central monoamines. The high level of glucocorticoid receptors on central monoamine neurones is postulated as mediating the alteration. There are two types of cortisol receptor in the mammalian brain: the type 1 receptor (or mineralocoticoid receptor)

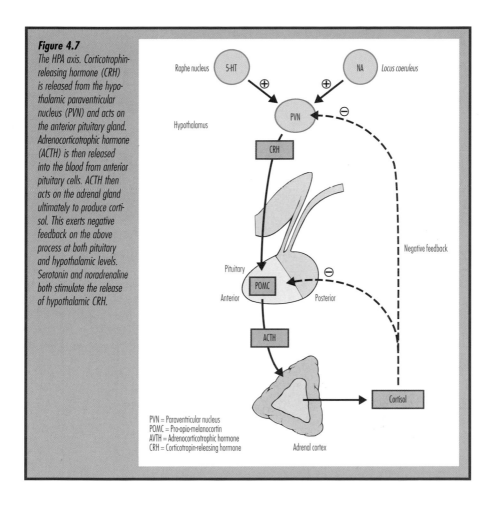

Figure 4.7
The HPA axis. Corticotrophin-releasing hormone (CRH) is released from the hypothalamic paraventricular nucleus (PVN) and acts on the anterior pituitary gland. Adrenocorticotrophic hormone (ACTH) is then released into the blood from anterior pituitary cells. ACTH then acts on the adrenal gland ultimately to produce cortisol. This exerts negative feedback on the above process at both pituitary and hypothalamic levels. Serotonin and noradrenaline both stimulate the release of hypothalamic CRH.

PVN = Paraventricular nucleus
POMC = Pro-opio-melanocortin
AVTH = Adrenocorticotrophic hormone
CRH = Corticotropin-releasing hormone

and the type 2 receptor (or glucocorticoid receptor). The former receptor is predominantly found in the septo-hippocampal projection. The type 2 receptor is distributed widely throughout the brain (especially in monoaminergic neurones), and it monitors stress elevations in cortisol. Both the serotonergic and noradrenergic

Receptor	Location	Actions
Noradrenergic α_1	Post-synaptic	Vasoconstriction — raises blood pressure
Noradrenergic α_2	Pre- and post-synaptic	Presynaptic autoreceptor regulates release of noradrenaline; pre-synaptic heteroreceptor regulates release of serotonin

Table 4.1
Noradrenergic receptors.

Receptor	Location	Actions
$5HT_1a$	Presynaptic/Autoreceptor*	Inhibits serotonin release, antidepressant action, anxiolytic action
$5HT_2a/c$	Post-synaptic	Antidepressant action Serotonin-mediated side-effects — anxiety, sexual dysfunction, insomnia
$5HT_3$	Post-synaptic	Gastrointestinal side-effects (nausea, diarrhoea)

* There is also a post-synaptic 5HT1a receptor.

Table 4.2
Serotonergic receptors.

neurones are influenced by cortisol. Traditionally, the monoamine abnormalities seen in depression have been regarded as primary. All current pharmacological interventions for depression are aimed at the monoamine system. It may, however, be more appropriate to view the monoamine abnormalities as secondary to disturbances in the HPA. Future generations of antidepressants may target the HPA rather than the monoamine system.[19] An example of such a strategy would be the current development of drugs which act as CRH receptor antagonists.

Key Points

- Family, twin and adoption studies have shown that there is a significant genetic component to depressive disorders.

- There are several lines of evidence for abnormal noradrenergic and serotonergic function in depressive disorders.

- Antidepressants cause various neurochemical changes; however, their specific antidepressant effects remain unknown.

- The neuroendocrine axis is often altered in depressive disorders and may be the mediator of environmental influences. Alternatively it may be the primary cause of depression in certain depressive sub-types.

References

1. Taylor MA, Berenbaum SA, Jampala VC. Are schizophrenia and affective disorders related? Preliminary data from a family study. *American Journal of Psychiatry* (1993) **41**: 949–58.

2. Bertelsen A, Harvald B, Gauge M. A Danish twin study of manic-depressive disorders. *British Journal of Psychiatry* (1977) **130**: 330–51.

3. Kendler KS, Neale MC, Kessler RC. A population based twin study of major depression in women: the impact of varying definitions of illness. *Archives of General Psychiatry* (1992) **49**: 272–81.

4. McGuffin P, Katz R. The genetics of depression and manic depressive illness. *British Journal of Psychiatry* (1989) **155**: 294–304.

5. Mendlewicz J, Rainer JD. Adoption study supporting genetic transmission in manic-depressive illness. *Nature* (1977) **268**: 327–9.

6. Wender PH, Kety SS, Rosenthal D. Psychiatric disorders in the biological and adoptive families and adopted individuals with affective disorders. *Archives of General Psychiatry* (1986) **43**: 923–9.

7. Cadoret RJ, O'Gorman TW, Heywood E. Genetic and environmental factors in major depression. *Journal of Affective Disorders* (1985) **9**: 155–64.

8. Berretini W. Genetic studies of bipolar disorders: new and recurrent findings. *Molecular Psychiatry* (1996) **1**: 172–3.

9. Calloway P, Dolan R. Endocrine changes and clinical profiles in depression. In: Brown GW, Harris TO eds, *Life Events and Illness* (London: Unwin Hyman, 1989) 139–60.

10. Gunnar MR, Larson MC, Hertsgaard L. The stressfulness of separation among nine-month old infants: effects of social context variables and infant temperament. *Child Development* (1992) **63**: 290–303.

11. Schildkraut JJ. The catecholamine hypothesis of affective disorders: a review of supporting evidence. *American Journal of Psychiatry* (1965) **122**: 509–22.

12. Coppen A. The biochemistry of affective disorders. *British Journal of Psychiatry* (1967) **113**: 1237–64.

13. Checkley SA. The neuroendocrinology of depression and chronic stress. *British Medical Bulletin* (1996) **52 (3)**: 597–617.

14. Stein JF. *An Introduction to Neurophysiology* (Oxford: Blackwell Scientific, 1982).

15. Stokes PE, Pick GR, Stoll PM. Pituitary-adrenal function in depressed patients: resistance to dexamethasone suppression. *Journal of Psychiatric Research* (1975) **12**: 271–81.

16. Nemeroff CB, Widerlov E, Bissette G. Elevated concentrations of CSF corticotrophin releasing factor-like immunoreactivity in depressed patients. *Science* (1984) **226**: 1342–4.

17. Dinan TG. Glucocorticoids and the genesis of depressive illness: a psychosocial model. *British Journal of Psychiatry* (1994) **164**: 365–71.

18. O'Keane V, McLoughlin D, Dinan TG. D-fenfluramine-induced prolactin and cortisol release in major depression: response to treatment. *Journal of Affective Disorders* (1992) **26**: 143–50.

19. O'Dwyer AM, Lightman SA, Marks MN. Treatment of major depression with metyrapone and hydrocortisone. *Journal of Affective Disorders* (1995) **33**: 123–8

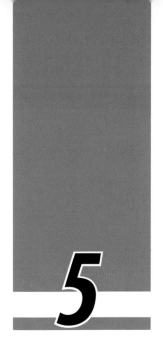

Physical treatments

5

Pharmacological treatment of depression

The potentially severe distress and disabilities caused by depression necessarily require that the illness be treated quickly and effectively, if only to avoid suicide. In addition to many psychological therapies, the availability of ever-increasing medications has made the management of depression more diverse and sophisticated but not necessarily more potent. It is important to note, however, that although many new antidepressants have been developed, there has been less of an advance in their efficacy and most improvements relate to their side-effect profiles. These aspects will be discussed focusing first on the issue of efficacy and then the individual characteristics and adverse effects of various groups of antidepressants. The use of antidepressants in pregnancy, breastfeeding and the extremes of age is considered in *Chapter 9* and the issue of toxicity in overdose is dealt with in *Chapter 10*.

For over a quarter of a century two main groups of antidepressants have featured in the treatment of depressive illness, namely, tricyclic antidepressants (TCAs) and monoamine oxidase inhibitors (MAOIs). The selective serotonin reuptake inhibitors (SSRIs) are relatively new and grew out of a suggested need for greater selectivity. A similar strategy, when applied to the noradrenergic system, produced antidepressants such as maprotilene. More recently, compounds with actions on both systems (noradrenergic and serotonergic) are being favoured even though it is not yet clear whether any of these drugs, selective or not, have any greater efficacy.

Imipramine was the first TCA to be discovered and is still the benchmark for comparison of efficacy. Based on its tricyclic structure a whole class of antidepressants was developed, many of which are still in use today.

The link between monoamine oxidase inhibition and antidepressant effect was first recognized with iproniazid. It was developed from isoniazid which was being investigated for the treatment of tuberculosis. The MAOIs have never been used as widely as TCAs, primarily because of their potentially dangerous side-effects, a problem that has only recently been addressed by the development of a reversible MAOI, moclobemide.

Efficacy

Clinically, even in moderately severe depressives (the group thought to respond best to antidepressants), the rate of improvement is only 70%. The actual effect of treatment is still less, as the placebo response is more than 30%. Studies have shown that 'endogenous' or major depression responds better to antidepressants than 'neurotic' depression and that this is true for both tricyclics and the newer antidepressants (SSRIs and related compounds). The latter do not have enhanced efficacy and may in fact be less effective than traditional antidepressants. However, this is a difficult interpretation to make, as the newer, better tolerated medications are probably prescribed to a wider range of patients, including those in whom antidepressants would not necessarily be of any discernible help. Hence the difference in efficacy may be partly due to inappropriate use.

The assessment of depression and its response to treatment requires accurate definition and measurement. Major depression, as described previously, is a syndrome of depressed mood with diminished interest and capacity for pleasure (anhedonia), lasting at least two weeks and producing significant social or occupational impairment. Assessment scales which have a bias for certain features of depression are poor instruments by which to measure clinical changes, particularly those produced by pharmacotherapy, and therefore perhaps scales which examine the essential aspects of depression such as mood, suicidal intent and psychomotor changes should be used. In this respect, the CORE system and the Montgomery–Asberg Depression Rating Scale are good measures.[1, 2]

Mild depression has a significant placebo response and a high rate of spontaneous remission. It benefits little from medication and, likewise, brief recurrent depressions also show minimal response to pharmacotherapy.[3] However, severe illnesses such as psychotic depression, although also having a poor response to tricyclics and a low placebo effect, do improve to some degree. Tricyclics are effective in a third of cases and much more so in combination with an antipsychotic, but better still is electroconvulsive therapy (ECT) which successfully treats more than two thirds of cases.

Atypical depression seems to respond best to MAOIs, which are also useful in depressed patients with additional symptoms of panic or anxiety. Hence, antidepressants are of considerable use in the treatment of many kinds of depression although some symptoms, especially those classed as 'neurotic', usually do not respond to medication.

The response to medication is complicated and varied, with some features improving more than others. The fact that the symptoms of depression remit in stages makes it difficult to identify a specific point of recovery. However, a delay in the response to antidepressant treatment is well recognised and is considered to be about 2-6 weeks for tricyclics and SSRIs and a little longer for MAOIs. Part of the reason for the delay in therapeutic response is the difficulty in assessing recovery and the inclusion of those that respond poorly in the recovered group.

Adverse effects

Antidepressants either belong to one of the three main groups or are related in some way to them or have totally unique characteristics and are described as novel or atypical. The groups are formed on the basis of structural or functional similarities and so adverse effects are largely shared, with some minor differences and idiosyncrasies between individual antidepressants. As most antidepressants are equally effective, prescribing choice depends chiefly on suitability and so the adverse effects of these drugs are of great significance. Compliance, tolerance and risk in overdose are important considerations and so the side-effect profile of individual antidepressants determines their popularity and use.

The TCAs and MAOIs were the first groups to be developed and are often referred to as the 'classical antidepressants', although the indications for their use have expanded beyond depressive illness to include, for instance, the treatment of anxiety disorders (imipramine), obsessional disorders (clomipramine) and chronic pain (amitriptyline). These traditional groups of antidepressants will be considered first.

Tricyclic antidepressants (TCAs) *(Table 5.1)*

The tricyclics are so called because of their three-ring structure *(Figure 5.1)*. Depending on the number of methyl groups attached to the side-chain nitrogen, they are described as tertiary (two methyl groups) or secondary (one methyl group) amines, and their properties differ accordingly. Tricyclic therapeutic effects stem from their ability to block the reuptake of noradrenaline and serotonin; secondary amines preferentially block the reuptake of noradrenaline, while tertiary amines mainly block the reuptake of serotonin. However, they also act as antagonists at muscarinic, histaminic (H_1) and α_1-adrenergic receptors producing predictable and well characterized side-effects. The anticholinergic effects (dry mouth, constipation, blurred vision and urinary retention) of tricyclics are extremely common although with secondary amines they are less severe. The side-effects tend to diminish with continued treatment, but if they persist or are particularly troublesome they can be remedied with simple measures. Sugarless sweets can alleviate the dry mouth and bethanecol can be used to reduce urinary hesitancy. However tricyclics are contraindicated in narrow-angle glaucoma and can produce confusion and delirium, especially in the elderly.

All the tricyclics, with the exception of protriptyline and perhaps imipramine, have a sedating effect which may be of benefit to those suffering from insomnia. Amitriptyline and trimipramine are particularly sedative. Generally, the tertiary amines are more potent and produce marked sedation, particularly on commencement. This can also be of benefit to those with pronounced concomitant

	Sedation	Cardiotoxicity	Anticholinergic side-effects	Comments
Amitriptyline†	+++	+++	+++	Mild analgesic properties
Imipramine	++	+++	+++	
Trimipramine	+++	+++	+++	
Clomipramine†	++	+++	++	Mainly 5HT activity and useful for obsessional symptoms
Desipramine	+	++	++	
Doxepin	+++	++	++	Avoid in breastfeeding
Dothiepin	+++	+++	++	
Nortriptyline	+	++	++	
Protriptyline	—	+++	++	No sedation
Amoxapine	++	+	++	DA antagonist
Lofepramine	+	+	+	Safer in OD

+ = Mild   ++ = Moderate   +++ = Marked   DA = Dopamine   OD = Overdose

† = Can be given intramuscularly and intravenously

Table 5.1
Adverse effects of TCAs.

anxiety, although the sedating effects can be troublesome if they extend beyond sleep into the next day. Particularly important is the effect on reaction time which in turn affects the ability to drive and operate machinery safely.

The cardiovascular effects of tricyclics include orthostatic hypotension (via α_1-adrenoceptor blockade) and cardiac conduction abnormalities. The postural changes in blood pressure can often cause dizziness and result in injury from falls.

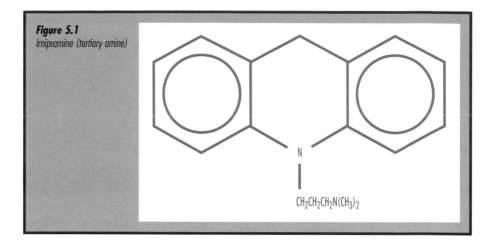

Figure 5.1
Imipramine (tertiary amine)

$CH_2CH_2CH_2N(CH_3)_2$

Again, secondary amines are less likely to have this effect and this is particularly true of nortriptyline. With overdoses, the direct effect of tricyclics on the heart can be fatal and, although cardiac contraction is probably not affected by tricyclics, they should not be used in patients with heart disease particularly with the advent of much safer drugs.

Other common side-effects of tricyclics are an increase in appetite (secondary to insulin activity) and weight gain (due to H_1 receptor blockade). In most severe depressives some weight gain is usually desirable. However, occasionally it can be a major problem and can limit treatment possibilities.

Tricyclics lower the seizure threshold and can thus induce fits, particularly in those predisposed. They should therefore be used with caution in those who suffer from seizures. Tremor is relatively common and two tricyclics, protriptyline and desipramine, are noted for their psychomotor stimulation.

Sexual dysfunction is a common problem but is often overlooked. Tricyclics can cause impotence and can also cause ejaculatory disturbances and anorgasmia. Much less common are idiosyncratic side-effects such as blood dyscrasias and hepatitis.

At extremely high blood levels, as in overdose, tricyclics bring about serious side-effects and can lead to death. High doses and adverse effects can also be the consequence of interaction with other drugs. Many SSRIs inhibit the metabolism of TCAs and can increase blood levels to the point of toxicity. MAOIs have an additive effect and can cause neuronal excitation and hypertension. These combinations are to be avoided.

From their side-effect profile, the interaction of tricyclics with anticholinergics, sedatives and cardiovascular drugs is readily predicted, producing a significant increase in the occurrence of adverse effects. However, whenever combining medications an appropriate formulary, such as the British National Formulary (BNF), should be consulted.[4]

The cessation of medication should be as careful as its commencement since withdrawal of long-standing tricyclic treatment can lead to symptoms of nausea, incontinence, seizures and confusion.

Monoamine oxidase inhibitors (MAOIs)
(Table 5.2)
Antidepressants in this group are defined by their ability to inhibit monoamine oxidase. Moclobemide is a selective and reversible inhibitor of MAO-A. The remaining so-called traditional MAOIs (phenelzine, tranylcypromine, isocarbox-

azid) are irreversible and produce very different adverse effects.

Anticholinergic effects and hypotension are dose-dependent adverse effects of the traditional MAOIs and, although common, with time they may diminish or even disappear. Other common effects are sedation and changes in weight. Of the traditional MAOIs, tranylcypromine is the least sedating and can actually act as a stimulant leading to insomnia. It is also thought to have addictive properties. However, it has less effect on weight than phenelzine which causes significant weight gain whereas isocarboxazid has, in some cases, been associated with weight loss.

Like the tricyclics, MAOIs can produce many forms of sexual dysfunction but, unlike the tricyclics, they do not lower the seizure threshold and are less cardiotoxic.

The MAOIs interact with many drugs (eg analgesics, antiepileptics, antidepressants), certain foods and general anaesthetics and they should therefore be stopped at least two weeks prior to any surgical operation.

Tyramine, which can act as a false noradrenergic neurotransmitter, is found in many foodstuffs and is normally metabolized by monoamine oxidase. If therefore

	Hypotension	Anticholinergic	Sedation	Notes
Isocarboxazid	+	+	+	Contraindicated in hepatic impairment or abnormal liver function tests
Phenelzine	+	+	+	
Tranylcypromine	+	+	—	Contraindicated in hyperthyroidism
Moclobemide	—	—	—	Contraindicated in acute confusional states
+ = Significant effect				

Table 5.2
Adverse effects of MAOIs.

ingested when its breakdown is inhibited, it can produce life-threatening hypertension. Consequently, several deaths have been reported and so when prescribing MAOIs it is essential to provide clear advice regarding food that can and cannot be eaten. It should be further noted that the traditional MAOIs can also interact adversely with sympathomimetics (eg ephedrine) and anorectics, producing a hypertensive crisis or a serotonin syndrome.

Moclobemide's reversible inhibition of MAO allows ingested tyramine to be metabolized. It therefore has fewer adverse effects and is better tolerated. The most common side-effects are nausea, dizziness, headache and insomnia. Restlessness and agitation occur infrequently and, exceptionally, moclobemide can cause confusion. To its advantage moclobemide prolongs sleep without REM suppression, unlike other MAOIs, and does not cause sexual dysfunction. Furthermore, it does not precipitate seizures or modify psychomotor performance and is therefore safe to use with epileptic patients.[5]

Moclobemide has few significant drug interactions, although with the SSRIs there is a risk of serotonin syndrome, and so this combination should be avoided.

Selective serotonin reuptake inhibitors (SSRIs) *(Table 5.3)*

The relatively new SSRIs have become popular due to their better tolerance and side-effect profile. The group has steadily expanded and now includes five agents, fluvoxamine, fluoxetine, paroxetine, sertraline and citalopram. SSRI-related side-effects are most prominent at the start of treatment and those most commonly reported are nausea, insomnia and anxiety-related symptoms. The latter, also termed activating symptoms, include perplexity, nervousness and agitation, and can be mitigated by the short-term use of benzodiazepines. In some individuals, rather than having an activating effect, the SSRIs lead to sedation and this, like the anticholinergic effects of these drugs, is most likely to occur with paroxetine. Sexual dysfunction, consisting of erectile failure in men, and reduced libido and anorgasmia in both sexes, is common and often leads to non-compliance. Like the other major groups of antidepressants, the SSRIs have many less frequent and idiosyncratic side-effects (for instance, rashes

	Sedation	Indications	Anticholinergic side-effects	Notes
Fluoxetine	—	BN, OCD	—	Long half-life; available as liquid
Fluvoxamine	+	OCD	—	Avoid in combination with theophylline
Paroxetine	+	OCD, panic disorder	+	Has withdrawal syndrome
Sertraline	—	Preventing relapse	—	Few known interactions
Citalopram	—	Panic disorder; preventing relapse	—	Few known interactions

+ = Significant effect   BN = *Bulimia nervosa*   OCD = Obsessive compulsive disorder

Table 5.3
Adverse effects of SSRIs.

and hair-loss) but, unlike the other groups, they do not cause weight gain. Overall, the SSRIs have few side-effects of less severity than the TCAs and the MAOIs. However, their interactions with other drugs can have serious consequences. The SSRIs inhibit a number of the hepatic cytochrome p450 enzymes and because of this they can increase the blood levels of other drugs metabolized by the same enzymes, such as the tricyclics. With MAOIs, the SSRIs cause the serotonin syndrome and so caution should be exercised when switching from one group of antidepressants to another.

Atypical antidepressants

Antidepressants that cannot be placed in any of the above groups are described as atypical or novel because of their unique pharmacology and mechanism of action. As a 'group' they are quite diverse and need to be considered individually.

Bupropion, (widely used in the USA), is a reuptake inhibitor of noradrenaline and dopamine. Its adverse effects, which mainly relate to changes of dopamine function, include nausea, agitation, weight loss, insomnia, seizures and psychosis. It is not sedative and does not possess anticholinergic or cardiotoxic effects, making it a useful alternative for tricyclics. However, its dose-dependent lowering of the seizure threshold requires that administration be carefully titrated.

Trazodone, is structurally related to the benzodiazepine alprazolam and acts as an antagonist at histaminergic and α_1-adrenergic receptors. It inhibits serotonin reuptake and has therefore an antidepressant effect. It is noted for its sedative effect in addition to which it commonly causes postural hypotension, dizziness, nausea and headache. It lacks anticholinergic effects and is less cardiotoxic than the tricyclics. It may cause priapism but this is a relatively rare complication. Trazodone should not be prescribed with MAOIs or SSRIs because of the danger of serotonin syndrome.

Nefazodone, is a potent $5HT_2$ receptor antagonist which inhibits both serotonin and noradrenaline reuptake and, like trazodone, blocks α_1-adrenoceptors. However, it has fewer side-effects than trazodone with a small proportion of patients complaining of nausea, sedation or occasional dizziness. Sexual dysfunction is rare and its use with epileptics seems to be safe, although it should still be administered with caution.[6]

Mianserin is a tetracyclic drug and an antagonist at pre-synaptic α_2-receptors and $5HT_2$ post-synaptic receptors. It acts as an antidepressant by disinhibiting noradrenergic transmission through α_2-autoreceptor blockade. Its actions at other receptors distinguish it from the tricyclics such that it has few anticholinergic effects and is much less cardiotoxic. Its most common adverse effect is that of sedation, which is usually mild and can often be beneficial in those with insomnia. It can also cause arthralgia, and there are reports of leucopenia and fatal agranulocytosis, which make regular blood monitoring a necessity. At present it is not available in the USA.

Mirtazapine, although only recently available in the UK, has been used for some time in Europe and USA. It is an antagonist at several receptors ($5HT_2$, $5HT_3$, H_1

and pre-synaptic α_2) and, by enhancing serotonergic and noradrenergic transmission, acts as a dual-action antidepressant. H_1 antagonism may lead to sedation and weight gain which in some cases can be desirable effects. Mirtazapine is also noted for its lack of nausea, agitation and sexual dysfunction due to $5HT_3$ and $5HT_2$ blockade. It lacks anticholinergic activity and is therefore better tolerated than the tricyclics. It also has a low propensity for drug–drug interactions as it neither inhibits nor induces hepatic enzymes.[7]

Venlafaxine is a reuptake inhibitor of both noradrenaline and serotonin. It is therefore a dual-action agent akin to standard tricyclics. However, it differs in that it has no cholinergic, histaminergic or α-adrenergic effects. Despite these differences it produces many dose-dependent adverse effects, some of which are similar to those produced by the SSRIs. Most noted is nausea which, although severe, is short-lived and can be treated by the use of cisapride. It occurs in approximately a third of cases and is often accompanied by somnolence, insomnia, headache, constipation, sweating or dry mouth. Agitation and anxiety are also frequently reported and so withdrawal from treatment is relatively common. In addition to the side-effects experienced at normal doses, at high doses venlafaxine can cause a sustained increase in blood pressure and so this should be closely monitored and its use in hypertensives avoided. Unlike most antidepressants, venlafaxine has few notable interactions and, unlike many of the newer drugs, it has a wide dosing range with corresponding gradation of efficacy.[8]

The clinical use of antidepressants is discussed in *Chapters 7, 8* and *9.*

Electroconvulsive therapy (ECT)

The clinical use of ECT depends upon the preferences of practitioners and patients, together with its perceived benefits and complications *(Table 5.4).* It was introduced in 1938 by Cerletti and Bini and has been in use ever since, although with the development of antidepressants it is less often used. However, it still has essential indications such as the treatment of severe resistant depression. Many comparisons of the two forms of therapy (ECT and antidepressants) have been carried out in order to define better their relative clinical indications and our understanding of their mechanisms of action. The efficacy, side-effects and clinical use of ECT have been extensively studied.[9–13]

ECT involves the application of electrical stimulation to the brain by passing a current between two electrodes placed in contact with the scalp. The patient is anaesthetized and their pulse, blood pressure and breathing are monitored. The seizure should ideally be monitored by EEG.

Table 5.4
Indications for the use of ECT in depression.

- Severe illness whereby patient refuses food and drink
- Psychotic depression
- Treatment resistance
- Previously responded to ECT
- Pharmacotherapy contraindicated

The stimulus-giving electrodes can be placed bilaterally or unilaterally and so two types of ECT can be prescribed. It should be noted that modified ECT does not produce any structural changes of brain matter, as assessed by sophisticated neuroimaging, and that ECT-induced seizures do not lead to neuronal death.[14, 15] The only absolute contraindication to ECT is raised intracranial pressure.

The presence of typical features of depression, in particular their severity and type, is the best predictor of recovery following ECT. Symptoms that show some specificity of response to ECT include depressive delusions, psychomotor retardation and intense suicidal preoccupation.[16]

The efficacy of ECT has been proven in comparison with simulated ECT and no treatment at all. Therapeutic effect is dependent upon the induction of a seizure which can be achieved by both unilateral and bilateral ECT. The latter is used more often in routine clinical practice and is given twice weekly (in the UK). In the USA bilateral ECT is given thrice weekly as standard and this is thought to have a faster onset of action.[17] Although this may have a quicker antidepressant effect and

can be used if speed of recovery is of particular importance, during the course of ECT it impairs cognition if given more than biweekly. In this respect unilateral ECT is much better than bilateral ECT as it produces less cognitive impairment. However, it is unclear whether it is as effective clinically, and a compromise utilizing both forms of ECT is probably best (bilateral ECT at beginning of course and then later switching to unilateral ECT) when concerned about cognitive impairment.[12, 18]

ECT is commonly and effectively used in the treatment of depression after antidepressants have been tried unsuccessfully. Although it is effective, the rate of recovery is probably slower than when used as a first-line treatment. It is unclear whether this is due to changes brought about by the prior use of antidepressants or simply that more treatment-resistant cases are included once one form of therapy has failed.[19] Like antidepressants, clinical improvement following ECT is delayed and, once achieved, it should be maintained by continuing treatment with antidepressants to prevent early relapse *(Table 5.5)*.

Table 5.5
Key points concerning ECT.

- Bilateral ECT preferred choice
- Preferably twice a week
- Optimum course: eight treatments or more
- Post-ECT confusion rarely > 1 hour
- Useful in elderly, even with comorbid dementia
- Unilateral ECT causes less cognitive impairment
- Establish antidepressant treatment to avoid relapse

Key Points

- Antidepressants are particularly effective in the treatment of moderate and severe depressive disorders. Psychotic depression requires the additional use of neuroleptics or alternatively ECT.

- With all antidepressants there is a delay in therapeutic effect. However, a lack of response should initially prompt reassessment of the diagnosis and adequacy of treatment.

- Clinically, almost all the various antidepressants are equally effective and significant differences exist only in their side-effect profiles. The suitability of an antidepressant is therefore dependent upon its interactions and adverse effects.

- The adverse effects of the main groups of antidepressants are summarised in **Tables 5.1, 5.2** and **5.3**. The key points concerning ECT are outlined in **Table 5.5**.

References

1. Parker G, Hadzi-Pavlovic D, Boyce P. Classifying depression by mental state signs. *British Journal of Psychiatry* (1990) **157**: 55–65.

2. Montgomery SA, Asberg N. A new depression scale designed to be sensitive to change. *British Journal of Psychiatry* (1979) **112**: 1165–71.

3. Paykel ES, Hollyman JA, Freeling P et al. Predictors of therapeutic benefit from amitriptyline in mild depression: a general practice placebo-controlled trial. *Journal of Affective Disorders* (1988) **14**: 83–95.

4. BMA and Royal Pharmaceutical Society of Great Britain. Drugs Acting on CNS. *British National Formulary*. No. 35 (1998) 155–232.

5. Stimmel GL, Dopheide JA. Psychotropic-induced reductions in seizure thresholds. *CNS Drugs* (1996) **1**: 37–50.

6. Robinson DS, Roberts DL, Smith JM. The safety profile of nefazodone. *Journal of Clinical Psychiatry* (1986) **57 (suppl 2)**: 31–8.

7. Davies R, Wilde M. Mirtazapine: a review of its pharmacology and therapeutic potential in the management of major depression. *CNS Drugs* (1996) **5**: 389–402.

8. Guelfi JD, White C, Hackett D et al. Effectiveness of venlafaxine in patients hospitalised for major depression and melancholia. *Journal of Clinical Psychiatry* (1995) **56**: 450–8.

9. Brandon S, Cowley P, McDonald C. Electroconvulsive therapy: results in depressive illness from the Leicestershire trial. *British Medical Journal* (1984) **288**: 22–5.

10. Gregory S, Shawcross CR, Gill D. The Nottingham electroconvulsive therapy study: a double-blind comparison of bilateral, unilateral and simulated ECT in depressive illness. *British Journal of Psychiatry* (1985) **146**: 520–4.

11. Greenblatt M, Grosser GH, Wechsler H. Differential response of hospitalised depressed patients to somatic therapy. *American Journal of Psychiatry* (1964) **120**: 935–43.

12. Sackeim HA, Prudic J, Devanand DP. Effects of stimulus intensity and electrode placement on the efficacy and cognitive effects of electroconvulsive therapy. *New England Journal of Medicine* (1993) **328**: 839–46.

13. Medical Research Council Clinical trial of the treatment of depressive illness. *British Medical Journal* (1965) **i**: 881–6.

14. Devanand DP, Dwork AJ, Hutchinson ER. Does ECT alter brain structure? *American Journal of Psychiatry* (1994) **151**: 957–70.

15. Scott AIF. Does ECT alter brain structure? *American Journal of Psychiatry* (1995) **152**: 1403.

16. Scott AIF. Which depressed patients will respond to electroconvulsive therapy? The search for biological predictors of recovery. *British Journal of Psychiatry* (1989) **154**: 8–17.

17. Rodger CR, Scott AIF, Whalley LJ. Is there a delay in the onset of the antidepressant effect of electroconvulsive therapy? *British Journal of Psychiatry* (1994) **164**: 106–9.

18. Sackeim HA, Decina P, Canzler M. Effects of electrode placement on the efficacy of titrated, low-dose ECT. *American Journal of Psychiatry* (1987) **144**: 1449–55.

19. Prudic J, Sackeim HA, Devanand DP. Medication resistance and clinical response to electroconvulsive therapy. *Psychiatry Research* (1990) **31**: 287–96.

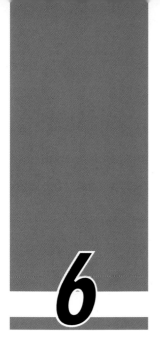

Psychosocial aspects of depression and psychological therapies

Introduction

In addition to the biological causes of depression it is now recognized that its multifactorial aetiology encompasses social and psychological factors. A research-based model bringing together the psychosocial aspects of depression has been developed and is shown diagrammatically in *Figure 6.1*. Most studies have involved populations of depressed women and have attempted to find links between early life experiences, the extent of social supports and the onset and maintenance of depression. The relationship between adversity and depression has been broken down systematically so as to allow description of its qualitative aspects. Crises that precipitate depression or cause a predisposition have been described as life events. These severe events involve the disruption of important social roles or are associated with experiences of defeat, entrapment and loss.

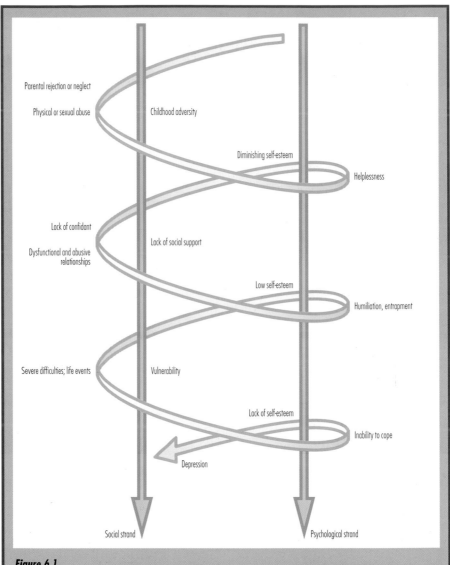

Figure 6.1
Psychosocial model of depression: illustrating the interaction of psychological and social elements.

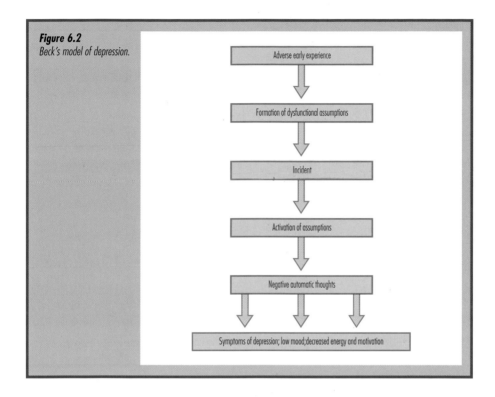

Figure 6.2
Beck's model of depression.

Adverse early experience

↓

Formation of dysfunctional assumptions

↓

Incident

↓

Activation of assumptions

↓

Negative automatic thoughts

↓ ↓ ↓

Symptoms of depression; low mood; decreased energy and motivation

Life events, adversity, hopelessness and entrapment

Major life events have serious negative implications and produce lasting change. Of these, some pose a significant threat over a lengthy period of time and seem to play a causal role in depression. There are two components of threat — loss and danger — that are important. Losses can be material, financial or the disruption of close relationships. These losses, if severe, may engender feelings of low self-esteem and humiliation which in turn may lead to hopelessness and entrapment.

The context of life events is also important as the same life event can have markedly different consequences, depending upon the circumstances of the individual concerned and how they deal with changes to their life. For instance, the birth of a baby is usually seen as a happy event and is likely to be a positive influence when the mother is wanting the baby and has support from family and friends. However, the same 'event' could be a significant negative influence if the child is unwanted or is seen as a burden. It is therefore necessary to note not only the changes that affect people's lives but also 'how' these changes take effect and what they mean to that particular individual in the context of their life.

Continuing problems causing chronic adversity are described as 'difficulties'. When severe and enduring, these 'major difficulties' can also lead to depression. It is noteworthy that the majority of those who experience a 'severe event' or have 'major difficulties' do not become depressed. This means that within some individuals there is a propensity for depression following an event or a series of difficulties, and it is this tendency that is termed 'vulnerability'.

Danger, the other component of threat, refers to possible future events that might result in loss or pose a specific risk of loss. It is more closely associated with the occurrence of anxiety disorders as opposed to depression. [1, 2]

Vulnerability factors, attachment and coping strategy

These are factors which, in the presence of major difficulties or following the occurrence of severe events, increase the likelihood of depression. They fall into two groups, psychological and environmental, and can collectively be referred to as psychosocial vulnerability factors.

Early research identified several factors, such as the lack of employment outside the home, the presence at home of three or more children (below the age of 15 years) and early maternal loss (before the age of 11 years), as predictors of depression. However, recent studies indicate that these are perhaps superficial markers of more central vulnerability factors pertaining to lack of social support and negative self-evaluation. [3, 4, 5]

The main psychological factors that have been closely associated with the onset of depression are low self-esteem, chronic anxiety and ongoing symptoms of depression, which are in themselves insufficient to make a diagnosis of depressive illness.

The other group of factors that generate vulnerability concern, in one form or other, deficits in emotional and social support. Of particular note are the lack of a confidant, particularly at times of stress or crisis. Problems in valued relationships reinforce negative self-evaluation and collectively create a vulnerable individual.

These vulnerabilities seem to be a consequence of childhood adversity. Studies of depressed women have shown that physical or sexual abuse during childhood or parental rejection or neglect tend to lead to dysfunctional relationships. Women with such experiences are more likely to have early pregnancies and unstable relationships with unreliable partners. These circumstances then predispose them to the vulnerabilities discussed, thus increasing their chances of depressive illness.

It is important to note that 'social support' is the synthesis of internal and external components, and that the internal component, concerning the individual's ability to relate and develop relationships, is no doubt crucial in determining whether external supports, if present, are utilized effectively. The manner in which these skills of relating to others are employed is broadly termed 'attachment style'.

Another matter that relates to the depressed individual's personality and behaviour is their style of coping. Following the occurrence of difficulties or events, the manner in which these are approached seems to play a determining role. Confronting the posed 'threat' and attempting to diminish its consequences by seeking some positive meaning is usually helpful, whereas dealing with the situation in a helpless and self-critical fashion increases the risk of depression.[6, 7]

Cognitive theory

Beck's cognitive theory for depression provides a model for understanding its development.[8–10] It postulates that certain 'core beliefs', concerning oneself and others, take form early in life. These are considered to be truths and are remembered as statements in simple sentences. Childhood experiences of adversity, such as rejection or abuse, help generate these core beliefs which then act as cognitive schemata. The latter are thought processes which follow basic rules and allow comprehension of the environment. Similarly, 'dysfunctional assumptions' which are modifications of the core beliefs are also schemata. The individual generates these so as to allow him or her to deal with their thoughts and beliefs. Cognitive vulnerability thus stems from this, particularly in relation to matters of acceptance, control, achievement and love. The fixed, uncompromising nature of these assumptions identifies them as dysfunctional and eventually when reality falls short of them they ultimately induce a sense of failure. Challenging these assumptions causes marked changes of emotion, and depressed mood is thought to arise when an individual's vulnerability is exposed, endangering their sense of self-worth. Once depressed the individual automatically develops negative thoughts relating to and perhaps reinforcing their dysfunctional assumptions. In this manner, once the symptoms of depression and negative cognitions are created, they maintain the illness.

Therefore, in Beck's model there are two main mechanisms that produce depression: the cognitive triad and errors of logic. The cognitive triad comprises three patterns of thought. The first is the individual's negative view of themselves, in which the individual believes that they are in some way defective or deprived and that this is because of a personal inadequacy of a psychological or physical nature. The second pattern concerns the individual's interactions with the world. Depressives tend to make negative interpretations of their experiences and therefore feel a sense of defeat and failure. The last component is the tendency to be pessimistic and hopeless about the future. The depressed individual expects continuing difficulty, suffering and failure, and holds no hope for improvement.

In Beck's model, errors in logic are generally followed by negative automatic thoughts. These appear spontaneously in the mind of the depressed individual and are therefore difficult to control. The fact that they are plausible also makes them difficult to challenge. They occur in response to all kinds of stimuli and eventually the patient develops negative reactions towards everything. Like obsessive thoughts, once a negative thought has emerged it is hard to dismiss. Errors of thinking support and confirm the patient's negative thoughts and beliefs and continue to occur despite cogent evidence to refute them. They are listed in *Table 6.1*.

Psychosocial model of depression

It is important to note that mood, behaviour and cognition are interconnected and affect each other, and that negative cognitions are part of the process of depression and are able to sustain depressed mood.

Overgeneralization — Evidence from a small number of events is inaccurately applied to a wider set of experiences, which may or may not be related, resulting in incorrect conclusions and interpretations

Catastrophic thinking — Extreme overgeneralization

Absolutistic thinking; dichotomous thinking; black-and-white thinking — Patient unnecessarily divides range of likely outcomes into polarized extremes and places self in negative categories

Selective abstraction — Positive or neutral information is disregarded and instead the patient recalls only undesirable and negative memories and events. The patient is said to have a selective negative focus and constructs their experience on the basis of less salient features taken out of context

Personalisation — The patient incorrectly interprets experiences as personally indicative of negative aspects of themselves

Arbitrary inference — The patient draws a particular conclusion in the absence of any supporting evidence or even when the evidence opposes the conclusion

Table 6.1
Cognitive distortions (errors of thinking).

Core beliefs and assumptions are forged from early experiences. Bowlby stressed the importance of secure attachment to a primary care-giver and suggested that this allows the development of independent, adult social functioning.[9] However, insecure attachment because of inconsistent care and rejection results in anxiety or avoidance. The implication, then, is that adverse childhood experience moulds an impression of the self and others which is subsequently used as a reference for future interactions and relationships. It is therefore assumed that individuals with attachment problems will, in the course of their life, experience difficulties within relationships.

Parents and their style of care are important influences in childhood. Parents contribute significantly to the injection of values, self-worth, expectations and attitudes, and so play a formative role in the creation of personality. Parenting style influences development, modifying personality to create vulnerabilities which, when impinged upon by incidents and events relating to acceptance, ability or love, lead to negative thoughts pertaining to the situation. This then leads to associated automatic thoughts, feelings and emotions which may culminate in symptoms of depression. These concepts and ideas have some support and provide a means of linking environmental influence and psychological processes. [11, 12]

Psychological therapies

Many types of psychological therapy are available and most are carried out by trained therapists. Those used in depression are listed in *Table 6.2* and briefly described. At present, one of the most popular therapies for the treatment of depression is cognitive therapy (cognitive behavioural therapy; CBT).

	Cognitive therapy	Psychodynamic therapy	Interpersonal therapy
Aetiology	Distorted cognitions; learnt negative thought processes	Childhood unresolved conflicts causing low self-esteem	A lack of significant social bonding; damaged interpersonal relationships
Aims and method of change	Identify negative cognitions and modify dysfunctional assumptions; to create mastery of thoughts	To gain insight into the defects of the mind (ego, superego) and rectify these to facilitate changes in personality	To improve communication skills and to solve interpersonal problems in important arenas of life (eg at home, at work)
Clinical aspects of therapy	Symptom focused; short duration; therapist actively involved; tailored to treating depression	Emphasis on intra-psychic phenomena; open-ended, unspecified duration; therapist is passive and impartial	Focus is more on inter-personal and environmental factors; duration is limited

Table 6.2
Psychological therapies used in depression.

Cognitive therapy

CBT involves identifying the patient's faulty thought processes. The patient is made aware of their 'negative automatic thoughts' and 'dysfunctional assumptions' and the therapist helps the patient to modify these by examining the events and reasoning that led to their development. Specifically, the therapist often questions the patient's logic so as to generate alternative patterns of thought. Typically, cognitive therapy involves a course of 12–20 sessions. Each session is structured jointly by therapist and patient. *(Table 6.3)*.

Between sessions, the patient is usually set 'homework', which is then examined by the therapist who normally takes a problem-orientated approach and plays an active role in directing therapy. Essentially, the therapist attempts to teach the patient various techniques and so initial sessions are more didactic. The patient is expected gradually to learn the various skills required to monitor their thoughts and test their assumptions in the future. There is a growing body of evidence that shows that cognitive therapy is effective in some depressive disorders.[13]

Psychodynamic therapy

Psychoanalysis attempts to reorganise a patient's personality. It is of lengthy duration with emphasis on intrapsychic phenomena. In contrast, psychodynamic therapy is brief and focused, whilst still utilising the principles of psychoanalysis.

1. Assessment of mood (Beck Depression Inventory)
2. Jointly decide on content of session
3. Review of events, feedback from previous sessions and discussion of homework
4. Main topic for discussion during this session
5. Summary of session with feedback and assignment of homework

Table 6.3
Contents of typical cognitive therapy session.

It aims to resolve unconscious conflicts and thereby treat depressive symptoms by facilitating comprehension of personal and interpersonal difficulties. The therapist interprets the patient's thoughts and behaviour, and through this process the patient attempts to gain insight into their emotional problems. Psychodynamic psychotherapy is effective in the treatment of certain depressed patients.[14, 15]

Interpersonal therapy

The premise in interpersonal therapy is that depressive symptoms arise in specific interpersonal contexts. These contexts need to be reexplored and understood and so the therapist, in addition to being supportive and understanding, is also quite active. Following an initial explanatory or educational stage, in which the patient's current social relationships are reviewed with a view to drawing out links to their illness, the therapist then pursues a specific interpersonal theme and uses strategies to resolve interpersonal difficulties. Therapy is eventually brought to a conclusion by appraising that which has been gained and by focusing on the prevention of depressive symptoms. Like cognitive and psychodynamic therapies, interpersonal therapy has been shown to be effective in depressives.[16, 17]

Key Points

- The psychosocial aspects of depression are important in both precipitating and maintaining depressive illnesses.

- Psychological interventions are often effective and usually more acceptable to the majority of patients.

- Psychological therapies need to be tailored to the needs of the patient and can normally be used in combination with pharmacotherapy.

References

1. Brown GW, Bifulco A, Harris TO. Life events, vulnerability and onset of depression: some refinements. *British Journal of Psychiatry* (1987) **150**: 30–42.

2. Paykel ES, Tanner J. Life events, depressive relapse and maintenance treatment. *Psychological Medicine* (1976) **6**: 481–5.

3. Brown GW, Harris TO. *Social Signs of Depression: A Study of Psychiatric Disease in Women* (New York: Tavistock Press, 1978).

4. Brown GW, Andrews B, Harris TO et al. Social support, self-esteem and depression. *Psychological Medicine* (1986) **16**: 813–31.

5. Brown GW et al. Self-esteem and depression. *Social Psychiatry and Psychiatric Epidemiology* (1990) **25**: 225–34.

6. Brown GW, Harris TO, Hepworth C. Loss, humiliation and entrapment among women developing depression: a patient and non-patient comparison. *Psychological Medicine* (1995) **25**: 7–21.

7. Craig TKJ. Adversity and depression. *International Review of Psychiatry* (1996) **8**: 341–53.

8. Beck AT, Rush AJ, Shaw BF et al. *Cognitive Therapy for Depression* (New York: Wiley, 1979).

9. Stern R, Drummond L. *The Practice of Behavioural and Cognitive Psychotherapy* (Cambridge: Cambridge University Press, 1991).

10. Moorey S. Cognitive therapy. In: Dryden W ed, *Individual Therapy. A Handbook* (Milton Keynes: Open University Press, 1995) 226–51.

11. Carnelley KB, Pietromonaco PR, Jaffe K. Depression, working models of others and relationship functioning. *J Pers Soc Psych* (1994) **66**: 127–40.

12. Bowlby J. *A Secure Base: Parent–Child Attachment and Healthy Human Development* (New York: Basic Books, 1988).

13. Gloaguen V, Cottraux J, Cucherat M et al. A meta-analysis of the effects of cognitive therapy in depressed patients. *J Affect Disord* (1998) **49**: 59–72.

14. Robinson LA, Berman JS, Neimeyer RA. Psychotherapy for the treatment of depression: a comprehensive review of controlled outcome research. *Psych Bull* (1990) **100**: 30–49.

15. Strupp HH, Binder JL. *Psychotherapy in a New Key: A Guide to Time-limited Dynamic Psychotherapy* (New York: Basic Books, 1984).

16. Klerman GL, Weissmann MM, Rounsaville BJ et al. *Interpersonal Psychotherapy of Depression* (New York: Basic Books, 1984).

17. Weissmann MM, Markowitz JS. Interpersonal therapy: current status. *Arch Gen Psych* (1994) **51**: 599–606.

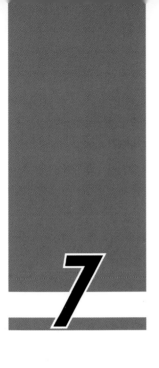

Management of depression in the community

The route by which depressed patients acquire a diagnosis and utilize healthcare services can be mapped against a framework devised by Goldberg and Huxley for individuals with mental illness.[1] In this there are five levels, each of which equates to a stage along the route of assessment and care. Movement from one level to the next entails passing through a filter, and there are four such filters which have to be negotiated successfully in order to gain access to the final level (specialized hospital services). *Figure 7.1* shows this in diagrammatic form. This chapter is mainly concerned with the first three levels and the two filters between them.

Depression in the community

Depressive disorders are by far the most common psychiatric illnesses encountered in the community. They are more prevalent in women, a difference which is less

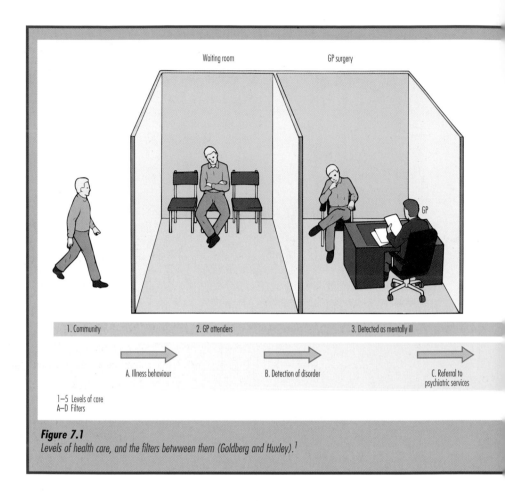

Waiting room   GP surgery

GP

1. Community   2. GP attenders   3. Detected as mentally ill

A. Illness behaviour   B. Detection of disorder   C. Referral to psychiatric services

1–5 Levels of care
A–D Filters

Figure 7.1
Levels of health care, and the filters betwween them (Goldberg and Huxley).[1]

marked in patients who have contact with mental health services, and are reported to occur in as many as a quarter of those consulting their GP.[2, 3]

Difficulties concerning the detection and diagnosis of depression are most evident in the setting of the community and general practice.[4] Many individuals,

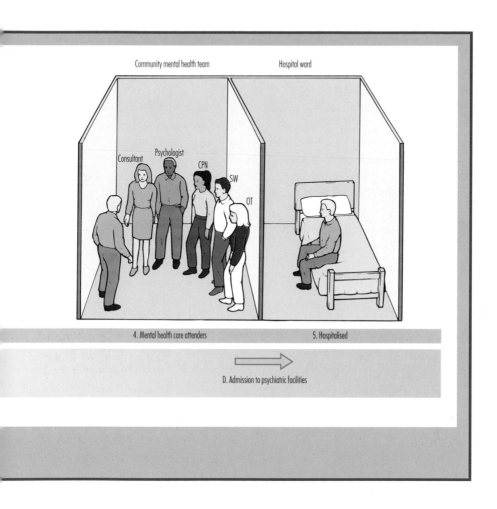

although they have a significant number of depressive symptoms, do not perceive themselves as being mentally ill, and instead seek help for somatic symptoms.

Presentation to GP

The majority of depressed individuals present to their GP with physical problems:

the most common complaint, occurring in almost a third of such patients, is that of pain. Fatigue and disturbed sleep are other relatively frequent somatic presentations of underlying depression.[5]

Of those individuals presenting to their GP with symptoms of depression, just over 50% are diagnosed as having a depressive illness. Almost half go unrecognized and although, of these cases, many are self-limiting and a few are subsequently detected, a significant proportion remain unwell and untreated. However, this is probably partly because of the constraints of assessment and the characteristics of both patients and GPs.[1]

Depression is less likely to be recognized in patients who are young, physically ill or those who somatize. The converse is true for patients who are white, female or middle aged.

GPs have a limited period of time for interview within which they must arrive at a diagnosis and then formulate a suitable management plan. Due to this lack of time in most consultations, once depression is suspected screening questions can be used to elicit symptoms and make a diagnosis. Inquiry about mood, interest

and energy should be sufficient to indicate whether there is a need for further exploration.

The issue of detection is important, since many depressed patients respond to anti-depressant treatment. However, it is of note that better detection only marginally improves outcome, if at all, in the absence of education and advice regarding the management of depression.[6]

A commonly held view is that most cases of depression in primary care are mild and self-limiting. However, it has been discovered that almost 10% of patients presenting with depressive symptoms have major depression and a somewhat smaller but significant number have dysthymia. Even with treatment, only a few patients recover completely and the majority fail to respond fully and so continue to suffer. In total, approximately 10% of those who are ill eventually become chronic cases posing a tremendous burden on primary care services.

Treatment of depression

More than 80% of the individuals presenting to GPs with psychological ailments are depressed, anxious or both and the usual precipitant for consultations is some kind of social adversity or physical complaint, so that the task facing a GP (that of attempting to disentangle the necessary symptoms to make a diagnosis) is both complex and difficult.

Within this complicated picture the depressive illness itself can be of differing types and varying severity. Furthermore, the patients themselves may not be prepared to accept a psychological diagnosis and may not be willing, therefore, to take any advice or treatment the doctor has to offer. Having negotiated these difficulties to arrive at a diagnosis, the GP then has to decide upon the further management of the patient. This may include the prescription of an antidepressant or use of psychological therapies, either alone or in combination. Alternatively, social factors may need to be addressed and, indeed, all these aspects have to be considered along with practical details such as who will provide these interventions. Naturally, the resources available will determine the type of care possible and, in this regard, the GP also has to decide when to seek advice and when to involve psychiatric services.[9]

Antidepressants

For those with moderately severe depression antidepressant treatment is clearly effective. However, GPs often attempt to treat depressive illnesses with sub-therapeutic levels of antidepressants and compliance with medication is usually poor, with most patients stopping treatment within the first few weeks of commencing therapy.[10] Patients usually refuse treatment because of concerns about addiction or the development of side-effects. Therefore, when starting treatment, it is necessary to inform patients of likely side-effects and to explain, as far as possible, the rationale of pharmacotherapy. In this respect, the better tolerated SSRIs should increase compliance and encourage patients to remain in treatment.

Psychological and sociological therapies

In primary care, psychological treatments that have been shown to have a significant therapeutic effect are cognitive therapy and 'problem-solving'. However, it is of note that, in the primary care setting, there is little to distinguish the therapeutic efficacy of psychological and pharmacological measures. Furthermore, assessments of sociological interventions have seldom been made, as it is difficult to quantify their effectiveness, even though they are likely to be of significant value.[11–14]

Currently, the most important issue concerning the management of depression in primary care is that of 'unmet need'.

To raise awareness, the Royal College of Psychiatrists launched the 'defeat depression' campaign in 1992 aimed at educating both the general population and health-care professionals in matters relating to depressive illness. The campaign emphasised the recognition and appropriate treatment of depression.[15] The impact of this campaign is currently being evaluated.

Key Points

- Depression is common in the community. Many GP attendees have a depressive disorder but almost half of these are unrecognised.

- Only 10% of those diagnosed as having depression are referred to a psychiatrist and so the majority of cases are treated by GPs.

- Somatization and physical illness decrease the likelihood of detecting depression particularly in relatively young individuals.

- A high index of suspicion and the use of relevant screening questions is likely to increase the detection of depressive disorders.

- When commencing pharmacotherapy it is necessary to warn the patient of possible side-effects and attempt to allay any anxieties concerning treatment so as to enhance compliance.

- A therapeutic antidepressant dose should be achieved and maintained for at least three weeks.

- Psychosocial interventions are often effective particularly in mild and moderate depressive illnesses.

References

1. Goldberg DP, Huxley P. *Common Mental Disorders: A Biopsychosocial Approach* (London: Routledge, 1992).

2. Freeling P, Tylee A. Depression missed or mismanaged in primary care. In: Montgomery S, Rouillon F eds, *Long-term Treatment of Depression* (Chichester: Wiley, 1992), 15–31.

3. Roberts A, Priest RG. Depression in the community. *Primary Care Psychiatry* (1995) **1**: 5–13.

4. Tylee A, Freeling P, Kerry S. Why do practitioners recognize major depression in one woman yet miss it in another? *British Journal of General Practice* (1993) **43**: 327–30.

5. Goldberg DP, Bridges K. Somatic presentation of psychiatric illness in primary care setting. *Journal of Psychosomatic Research* (1988) **32**: 137–44.

6. Tylee A, Freeling P. The recognition, diagnosis and acknowledgement of depressive disorder by general practitioners. In: Herbst K, Paykel E eds, *Depression: An Integrative Approach* (Oxford: Heinemann, 1989).

7. Freeling P, Rao BM, Paykel ES et al. Unrecognised depression in general practice. *British Medical Journal* (1985) **290**: 1880–3.

8. Blacker CVR, Clare AW. Depressive disorder in primary care. *British Journal of Psychiatry* (1987) **150**: 737–51.

9. Rihmer Z, Rutz W, Pihlgren H. Depression and suicide in Gotland. An intensive study of all suicides before and after a depression-training programme for general practitioners. *Journal of Affective Disorders* (1995) **35**: 147–52.

10. Johnson G. Treatment compliance in general practice. *Acta Psychiatrica Scandinavica* (1981) **63 (suppl 209)**: 447–53.

11. Mynors-Wallis LM, Gath DH, Lloyd-Thomas AR. Randomised controlled trial comparing problem solving treatment with amitriptyline and placebo for major depression in primary care. *British Medical Journal* (1995) **310**: 441–5.

12. Ronalds C, Creed F, Stone K et al. Outcome of anxiety and depressive disorders in primary care. *British Journal of Psychiatry* (1997) **171**: 427–33.

13. Scott C, Tacchi MJ, Jones R et al. Acute and one-year outcome of a randomised controlled trial of brief cognitive therapy for major depressive disorder in primary care. *British Journal of Psychiatry* (1997) **171**: 131–4.

14. Teasdale JD, Fennell MJV, Hibbert GA et al. Cognitive therapy for major depressive disorder in primary care. *British Journal of Psychiatry* (1984) **144**: 400–6.

15. Paykel ES, Priest RG. Recognition and managment of depression in general practice: a consensus statement. *British Medical Journal* (1992) **305**: 1198–202.

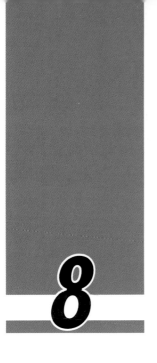

Hospital management of depression and resistant depression

8

Introduction

Hospitalization is indicated when depression poses a significant risk of self-harm, with severe anorexia or incapacitating symptoms. The decision to admit a depressed patient is to a large extent dictated by local and individual factors (resources available in the hospital, support available to the patient in the community from family, friends and healthcare professionals) and may involve compulsory detention. Patients can also be admitted for further investigation, or for more complex therapeutic interventions to be implemented.

On admission the patient's therapeutic history should be comprehensively reassessed. The aetiology of the illness should be considered taking into account psychological and social factors. It is also important to ask 'why now?' — that is, what, if anything, has precipitated this particular episode? Major depression, in particular, may not have external causes.

In addition to physical treatments such as medication and ECT, hospital admission provides immediate access to occupational therapy, psychological and psychotherapeutic interventions and the opportunity for patients to share the burden of the illness both formally in groups and informally in the ward milieu.

The principles of assessment and investigation of a depressed patient have been discussed in **Chapter 3**. The aim of this chapter is to review the treatment of depressive illness as encountered in psychiatric hospitals, focusing largely on pharmacological strategies. Many of these strategies are well established and widely used. However, some are only followed in specialist centres.

Initial choice of antidepressant

Depressive illness can be divided into several subtypes, namely, major and minor depression, dysthymia, psychotic depression and brief recurrent depression (see **Chapter 2**). Differentiation of depression on the basis of severity, duration and symptomatology is useful because these subtypes can sometimes be correlated to aetiological and prognostic factors.

However, research thus far has not been able to show satisfactorily whether these clinical subtypes of depressive illness differ therapeutically. The pharmacological specificity of different depressive subtypes can only be assessed convincingly through extensive clinical trials. In the absence of such information the initial choice of antidepressant is somewhat arbitrary and is dependent on some subjective (physician's preferences and experience) and objective factors (age, gender, comorbidity and past psychiatric history).

Specifically, there is no 'correct choice' of initial antidepressant and so treatment strategies will be discussed commencing with either a TCA or an SSRI. However, it should be noted that there is some evidence to suggest that TCAs are better suited to the treatment of severe depressive illnesses and that MAOIs, such as moclobemide, are most useful in atypical depression.[1]

As described in **Chapter 2**, ICD-10 divides depressive illness into mild, moderate and severe depression. The presence of psychotic symptoms creates a further diagnosis, namely, psychotic depression, and this will be discussed separately. Both mild and moderate depression warrant antidepressant pharmacotherapy, and treatment strategies are essentially the same, although mild depression has a significant placebo response and can often be treated with anxiolytics or neuroleptics.

In some instances, the antidepressant can be chosen on the basis of its side-effects — for instance, sedation or changes of appetite and weight may be of benefit in those with poor sleep or anorexic weight loss. However, if there is a significant risk of suicide, some of the newer antidepressants are perhaps more suitable.

Initially, a therapeutic dose of antidepressant should be achieved by titrating the prescribed dose against incipient side-effects and therapeutic response. Once an effective dose is accomplished it should be maintained for a period of at least three weeks, during which time it is important to ensure compliance and to monitor the patient closely for possible side-effects and signs of toxicity. If during this time there is some clinical improvement (partial response) then treatment can be continued at the same dose for a further three weeks. However, if after the initial three weeks there has been no clinical response, then the antidepressant dose should be increased. If despite this there is no clinical effect then it is best to consider either changing the antidepressant to one from a different class, preferably with a different mechanism of action, or attempting to augment the action of the antidepressant by adding an appropriate augmentor (see later). If either strategy fails — that is, switching or augmenting — then the other can be employed *(Figure 8.1)*.

From clinical experience, severe depression, as described by standard classifications or that which scores high on depression scales such as the HAM-D (> 25) or MADRS (> 30), seems to respond better to TCAs, and so these should be used in the first line of treatment.[2] Subsequently, the same strategy as for mild or moderate depression applies (switching or augmenting), except that treatment should commence at higher doses and consequently be monitored more closely. Patients with severe depression are invariably more functionally impaired and are at risk of developing medical complications due to inanition. Therefore, if pharmacotherapy fails ECT should be considered as the next line of treatment and in some cases it may be the initial treatment of choice (see *'Psychotic depression'* below).

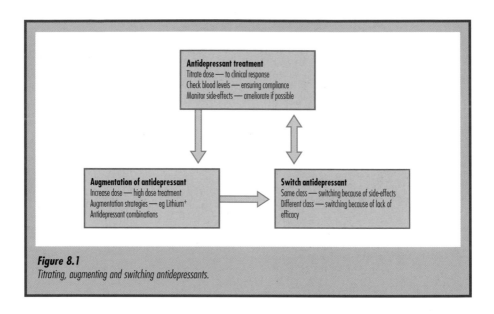

Figure 8.1
Titrating, augmenting and switching antidepressants.

Switching antidepressants *(Figure 8.2)*

If treatment with either a TCA or an SSRI fails, then switching between these two classes of drugs may help. Alternatively treatment can be switched from either of these groups to moclobemide or one of the novel antidepressants. It is noteworthy that often the change from one antidepressant to another is necessitated not by lack of efficacy but due to the occurrence of side-effects.

When changing antidepressant medication it is necessary to maintain an adequate 'washout period', during which antidepressant treatment is stopped so as to minimize the risk of drug interactions. This is particularly important when substituting with MAOIs. For most antidepressants (SSRIs and TCAs), three weeks is an adequate washout period before commencing treatment with an MAOI. However, in the case of fluoxetine double this period is required.

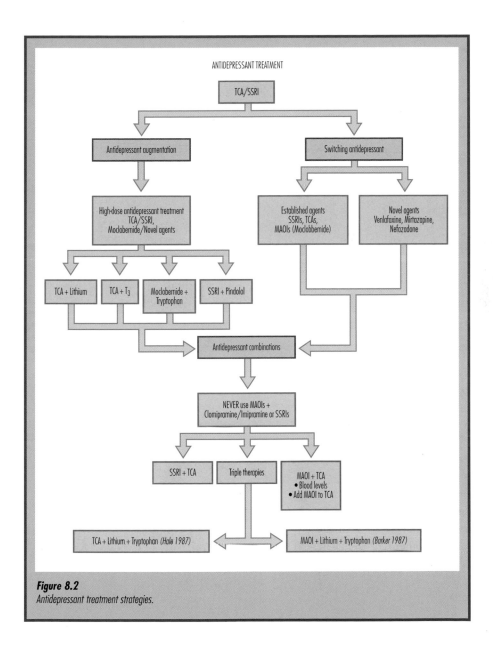

Figure 8.2
Antidepressant treatment strategies.

Switching between different classes of anti-depressants is often efficacious. However, within a particular class of antidepressants a different drug should only be considered if treatment has been inadequate due to the development of side-effects.[3]

Augmentation *(Figure 8.2)*

Lithium

It has been convincingly shown that the addition of lithium enhances the antidepressant effect of all three groups of antidepressants (TCAs, SSRIs and MAOIs). However, the addition of lithium poses difficulties as it has many potential side-effects and can interact adversely with SSRIs and MAOIs to produce the serotonin syndrome.[4] Therefore, having ensured that the patient has good thyroid and renal function, lithium should be added gradually with close supervision of its blood level so as to avoid toxicity. To attain a therapeutic effect, which may occur within a matter of days, lithium has to be administered at normal doses to give levels of 0.4–0.8 mmol/l.[5] If, initially, lithium augmentation produces a positive

response it is likely to remain effective in the long-term.[6] However, if the addition of lithium is ineffective then there are several alternatives, depending upon the antidepressant already in use.

The antidepressant effect of TCAs can be enhanced by the addition of T_3, that of SSRIs by the addition of pindolol, and that of MAOIs by the addition of tryptophan.

T_3

The addition of T_3 (triiodothyronine) to TCA treatment has been shown to be helpful in some cases of depression and, although abnormalities of the thyroid axis are associated with depressive disorders, the strategy is effective in euthyroid patients.[7–9] T_3 is more effective than thyroxine. However, T_3 augmentation is less predictable than the addition of lithium and can cause cardiac arrhythmias and agitation.

Pindolol

Negative feedback from intrasynaptic 5-HT via 5-HT$_{1A}$ autoreceptors inhibits serotonin release. Pindolol is an antagonist at 5-HT$_{1A}$

autoreceptors and therefore enhances serotonergic neurotransmission. Clinically, pindolol has been shown to be a useful adjunct enhancing the antidepressant effect of SSRIs and perhaps accelerating their speed of onset.[10,11] Unlike lithium the effect seems to be selective as pindolol does not augment the actions of other classes of antidepressants. Pindolol is also an antagonist at β_1-adrenoceptors. However, at the doses used (2.5 mg three times a day), it has little effect on these receptors, despite having a greater affinity for them than for 5-HT receptors. Since its mechanism of action is not completely understood, pindolol augmentation of SSRIs should be instituted with caution, noting also that it often causes marked sedation.

Tryptophan

The addition of tryptophan amplifies the antidepressant response of MAOIs. As described in **Chapter 4**, tryptophan is the amino acid precursor for serotonin and in combination with an MAOI enhances serotonergic neurotransmission in the brain. A contaminant of tryptophan manufacture, thought to have caused the eosinophilia-myalgia syndrome associated with its clinical use, led to its temporary withdrawal.[12] At present its prescription is limited to hospitals and the patient has to be registered for close haematological monitoring. Tryptophan has also been used in combination with clomipramine and lithium (see below) for the treatment of depression.[13]

Antidepressant combinations (Figure 8.2)

It is important to note that combinations of drugs, in addition to offering therapeutic advantages, can augment adverse effects and produce dangerous interactions.

Combinations of TCAs and MAOIs have been successfully used for many years.[14] However, it is essential to avoid the use of the tricyclics, imipramine and clomipramine, as they may cause fatalities, especially in combination with tranylcypromine.[15, 16]

Treatment should be started carefully, monitoring cardiovascular measures, and preferably adding a small dose of an MAOI to ongoing tricyclic treatment. Alternatively both drugs can be commenced simultaneously, again initially at low doses. The addition of a TCA to MAOI treatment is not recommended as it is even more likely to cause adverse effects.[17]

In a severely depressed patient, the combination of these drugs can be seen as a transitional stage when switching from a TCA to an MAOI, ensuring that the patient is never at any time without treatment. The side-effects of combining a TCA and an MAOI are essentially no different from those of the individual drugs. However, shared side-effects, such as anticholinergic side-effects, may become more pronounced. The efficacy of this combination has not been thoroughly evaluated and, given the development of new drugs, it is of limited use even in severe resistant depression.

SSRIs have been used in combination with TCAs. However, the efficacy of this strategy is not yet clear and most studies have been retrospective.[18] Clinically, the combination may produce a more pronounced antidepressant effect with faster onset. The addition of an SSRI to a TCA results in elevating the level of the latter due its displacement from protein binding sites and also because of inhibition of the cytochrome p450 system. This system is responsible for metabolizing TCAs and so when adding an SSRI the blood levels of antidepressants should be monitored, especially as most of the side-effects that ensue are due to raised levels.[19]

In almost a third of depressive episodes the use of an additional strategy, of either switching the antidepressant or augmenting it in some manner, will be necessary. However, a small number of patients require further measures such as a combination of antidepressants, high-dose treatment, or ECT. In these patients some novel strategies have been deployed and these will be discussed, along with the management of resistant depression.

Psychotic depression

Many would accept that psychotic depression has characteristics that differ from depression without psychotic features. Indeed, some would suggest that it is a distinct syndrome.[20] The clinical features of psychotic depression have been discussed in *Chapters 1* and *2*.

Approximately one sixth of patients with psychotic depression recover with treatment and remain well for a period of one year.[21] The majority (50–90%) relapse and the illness runs a recurring course.[22, 23] Antidepressants alone are only effective in a third of those with psychotic depression whereas, in combination with a neuroleptic, up to 80% of patients are likely to respond.[24] Thus far TCAs have been favoured because few other antidepressants have been used or assessed in the treatment of this disorder. SSRIs have been shown to be effective and are in some ways better suited as they are generally better tolerated and they elevate the plasma levels of concomitant neuroleptic medication.[25, 26] However, as SSRIs can also cause some extrapyramidal side-effects they can add to and exacerbate those produced by neuroleptics. Alternatively, because suicide is a greater risk in psychotically depressed patients, the relative safety of SSRIs in overdose is an important consideration.[27]

Maximum doses of all medications (neuroleptics and antidepressants) may be required and in some cases augmentation strategies similar to those already described may be necessary. The traditional neuro-leptics, if ineffective, may be substituted with novel or atypical agents such as clozapine, olanzepine, or risperidone, which have an additional effect on the serotonin system, or sulpiride, which has an antidepressant effect at low doses (100 mg/day).[28, 29] Once the patient has recovered the neuroleptic can be gradually stopped to minimize the risk of tardive dyskinesia, but given the high risk of relapse and recurrence, the antidepressant should be continued and perhaps maintained in the long term.

ECT should be considered early in the treatment of psychotic depression as it is very effective even in those patients who have failed to respond to antidepressant–neuroleptic combinations. In some cases it is perhaps the first treatment of choice, especially when the patient is known to have responded in the past and is resistant to pharmacotherapy.[30]

Resistant depression

Diagnosing resistant depression is dependent upon the assessment of symptoms and previous treatment. Definitions have been difficult to establish due to uncertainty concerning the adequacy of prior treatments.[31] Often resistant depression is secondary to physical illness or coexistent with other psychiatric disorders which complicate treatment. It is important therefore to exclude other diagnoses and explore the possibility of comorbidity. In addition to medical illnesses, such as thyroid disease or Cushing's syndrome, resistant depression may occur alongside anxiety disorders, obsessive compulsive disorder, personality disorder, and the abuse of alcohol or other drugs.

It is necessary to assess treatment resistance by evaluating the adequacy of all psychological and physical interventions. Even with severe depressive illnesses psychological treatments should not be overlooked as many patients are likely to benefit from formalized therapies such as cognitive behavioural therapy (CBT), and these can be readily administered at the same time as physical treatments.

The assessment of prior antidepressant and ECT treatment requires that both the administration of treatment and the response to treatment be examined. Issues of compliance, adequacy of dose, the need for therapeutic drug monitoring and the

duration of treatment as discussed in *Chapter 3* should be explored, checking that an appropriate treatment strategy has been followed in a systematic manner.[32]

A course of bilateral ECT should consist of at least eight applications of an adequate stimulus, producing seizures that are monitored and recorded, ideally, by EEG.[33] There is some debate about what is an adequate stimulus but most authorities agree that concerning bilateral ECT, a stimulus that is twice the threshold, or one which is achieved by titrating against seizure duration, is probably sufficient.[34] Another alternative is to use a fixed high-dose stimulus, although this is more likely to cause memory impairment. If these methods have not been used or if ECT has either been only unilateral or stopped prematurely, then the treatment has been inadequate and another course of ECT should be considered.

Some treatment strategies for resistant depression are used predominantly in specialist centres and these are summarized in *Table 8.1*. In some cases once all reasonable treatments have been tried unsuccessfully, then psychosurgery may be an option.[35] The latter is only available in a few centres around the world.[36]

Treatment	Notes	References
High-dose antidepressants	Particularly tricyclics, MAOIs and venlafaxine; blood levels are essential	Hodgkiss et al. 1995[37] Guze et al. 1987[38] Nierenberg et al. 1994[39]
Triple therapies TCA + lithium + tryptophan MAOI + lithium + tryptophan	Serotonin potentiation	Hale et al. 198[13] Barker et al. 1987[40]
DA agonists eg bromocriptine, pergolide	Reported efficacy in cases of resistant depression and as augmentors	Bouckoms and Mangini. 1993[41] Potter and Manji. 1994[42]

Table 8.1
Resistant depression treatment strategies.

Key Points

• The initial choice of antidepressant is dependent upon the characteristics of the depressive illness and those of the prescriber.

• Antidepressant dose should be titrated against clinical response and the development of side-effects. Where possible blood levels should be monitored and side-effects treated.

• Antidepressant effect can be augmented by either increasing the dose of medication or adding other treatments. The most widely used strategy is the addition of lithium.

• Switching antidepressants both within and between classes is a useful strategy if used appropriately.

• Psychotic depression is best treated with ECT or a combination of an antidepressant and antipsychotic.

• Resistant depression requires specialist treatment.

solely on the basis of signs and symptoms — regardless of whether they are due to a physical or psychological illness — could lead to overestimation. Diagnostically, depressive symptoms that are less likely to arise as a consequence of physical illness should be given greater importance *(Table 9.1)*. However, many doctors adopt the attitude that, in the context of a physical illness, psychological disorders are to some extent 'understandable'. This is an incorrect and unhelpful assumption that hinders the detection of depression as not all patients with physical illnesses become depressed, and those who do can often be successfully treated.

The degree to which physical illness determines the extent of any depressive disorder is dependent on several factors. The severity of the physical illness, although important, is not as significant a factor as one would anticipate. However, characteristics of the physical illness, such as the extent of pain due to disease or treatments and the patient's personality (in terms of style of coping and ability to do so) are significant determining factors.

Depression in physical illness has several consequences. It worsens the prognosis of some physical disorders and interferes with treatment by reducing enthusiasm for and compliance with medication.[4] Physically ill patients with depression have a reduced life expectancy and are less motivated and less likely to engage in therapeutic activities. Therefore treatment of the depressive illness allows better management of the physical illness and improves the individual's quality of life. Conversely, physical illnesses can exacerbate depressive disorders and can sometimes precipitate a depressive episode.

When presenting in the general hospital setting, depression in physical illness is usually assessed by a liaison psychiatrist;

Table 9.1
Depressive symptoms of diagnostic significance in physical illness.

- Guilt
- Worthlessness
- Anhedonia
- Hopelessness
- Unreactive mood

in the community it is managed largely by general practitioners. Some aspects of the assessment of depression are different because of the presence of a physical illness, and these are considered next.

A patient with a physical illness may feel that questions concerning their mental state undermine the importance of their physical symptoms and so it is appropriate initially to review these. However, the psychological implications of any changes should be borne in mind and explored carefully, in particular the effect the physical illness has on the daily activities of living. The patient's understanding and knowledge of the physical illness should be assessed since the patient may be unaware of the true nature of their illness, or there may be denial. Following this the cognitive symptoms of depression should be sought and the risk of suicide carefully gauged.

If a depressive illness is discovered, it should be treated promptly with due consideration of the various possible causes. If it is due to a physical illness, such as hypothyroidism, then it is this that needs to be treated. Similarly, if the depressive symptoms are a consequence of pharmacotherapy, this needs to be rationalized. The indications for the use of antidepressants or ECT remain the same, but the use of particular treatments is determined by the nature of the physical illness *(Table 9.2)*.

Generally, tricyclics are the preferred choice (provided they are not contraindicated) as they are reasonably well tolerated, cost-effective and analgesic.[5] The SSRIs can be used where there is a significant concern about suicide and the MAOIs should be avoided because of their complex pharmacological interactions.[6]

Treatment	Contraindicated use
TCAs	Liver/renal failure; recent myocardial infarct; acute glaucoma; agranulocytosis
MAOIs	Cardiac failure; cerebrovascular accident; hyperthyroidism
Lithium	Hypothyroidism; Addison's syndrome; renal failure

Table 9.2
Treatments and their contraindications.

Psychological intervention has been shown to be effective in some cases, as long as the therapy is focused, initiated early, and of relatively short duration.[7] Most therapies aim to improve the patient's quality of life by educating the patient about their physical illness and helping the patient to adapt to limitations and disabilities. Cognitive behavioural therapy and problem-solving are useful in these circumstances.

Depression in childhood and adolescence

Assessment and diagnosis

Childhood depression is relatively common both as a symptom and a disorder.[8, 9] The diagnosis of depression can be made using DSM-IV or ICD-10 definitions and the criteria for children are essentially the same as those for adults except that depressed mood can present as irritability and some of the criteria concerning the duration of illnesses are different — for instance, dysthymia need only be present for one year as opposed to two. Ideally, a variety of informants should be interviewed and all the information collated to produce a comprehensive picture of the illness.

Academic and social pressures at school are often overlooked, and so these should be investigated by gaining the relevant information from the pupil's teachers. Physical health is another important influence and, with the onset of puberty — particularly in girls — there is an increase in the likelihood of depressive symptoms.

In practice, comorbidity is the norm and this makes the treatment and management of depressive illness more complex. The most common comorbid conditions are anxiety and conduct disorders which coexist in about half of all cases of depression. The frequency of comorbidity is far greater than would be expected by chance, although it is possible that these high rates of comorbidity are in fact artifacts of poor classification.

Child and family characteristics

In pre-pubertal children, depression is slightly more common in boys, but this is reversed in adolescence and, by the mid-teens, the typical adult distribution of 2:1 in favour of females is attained. The families of depressed children have a greater preponderance of depressive disorders and alcoholism. However, the likelihood of depression within the family is only greater if the child is suffering from a depressive illness that has biological features, as opposed to one that is associated with conduct disorder. This familial tendency for disorders of mood is probably a function of both biological and environmental influences and underscores the need for thorough assessment of family members when managing depression in children.

Treatment

Decisions concerning the management of a child are best undertaken collectively involving, as appropriate, both family members and healthcare professionals (eg psychiatrists, general practitioners, psychologists and social workers).

Setting
The majority of depressed children are treated as out-patients as this maintains the child's 'natural' environment. In-patient treatment becomes necessary if the depressive illness disrupts schooling, impairs routine functioning and puts the child at risk of self-harm. Hospital admission is also advisable when starting medication and, occasionally, it is necessary for the management of associated

disorders, such as anorexia nervosa or drug abuse. In-patient treatment also allows more contact with the child and family members and enables close supervision of treatment. However, it may interfere with the child's long-term psychological development and should therefore be used with circumspection.

Treatment interventions
In the management of children's disorders it is quite usual to use several methods of treatment concurrently. Psychological therapies, pharmacological treatments and sociological interventions are therefore combined to address the needs of the child and family as a whole. In most cases, psychological treatment is most likely to be first line, particularly cognitive behavioural therapy which is widely practised and has been shown to be effective.[10] Other, less directed, forms of therapy, such as counselling, are not as effective, and depressive disorders that fail to respond to psychological therapy can be treated with antidepressants.

Childhood depressions that have marked biological features and a family history of depression are more likely to do well with pharmacotherapy. Initially, it is probably best to prescribe SSRIs as these are safer in overdose and have fewer side-effects than the TCAs. Furthermore, the TCAs have failed to show significant efficacy in childhood depression, although it should be noted that, in this age group, studies examining the efficacy of antidepressants are sparse and that the response to placebo is relatively high.[11] Following a therapeutic response, the possibility of relapse is also high (40% in two years), and so pharmacological treatment should be maintained for at least six months or more.

Implications and outcome
Childhood depression is a good predictor of suicide, and the involvement of psychiatric services enables the recruitment of many resources. Therefore, the management of childhood depression should involve an appropriate specialist child psychiatry team.

The occurrence of childhood depression increases the chances of depressive illness as an adult, and this should be borne in mind when discussing the long-term implication.[12] Furthermore, although most depressive illnesses in this age group resolve within a year, relapse is quite probable and so some degree of psychological intervention should be maintained to support and encourage recovery.[13]

Depression in the elderly

The diagnosis and treatment of depression are modified by age because of the biological and psychosocial changes associated with ageing.

Diagnosis

The elderly manifest depression differently, tending to under-report and diminish the importance of their feelings of sadness.[14] They often somatize, presenting with pain, but are also more likely to be suffering from a physical illness. The abrupt onset of anxiety is a common presentation and neurotic symptoms in general are most likely to be due to an underlying depressive illness.[15] Changes in behaviour can also be manifestations of depression, such that elderly depressives may become aggressive and threatening, or do the opposite, becoming withdrawn and refusing food. The onset of such behaviour usually coincides with changes in the social environment, for example moving into a nursing home.[16] In these instances collateral information is essential, and a knowledgeable informant should be actively sought.

Depression can also present with apparent symptoms of dementia, in particular memory deficits, and this is occasionally described as 'depressive pseudodementia'. Clinically, differentiating this from true dementia is often difficult, although the onset of cognitive impairment due to depressive illness can usually be specified by informants, and the patients themselves are aware of memory problems and complain repeatedly. However, when tested, they are more prone to become irritated and reply 'don't know' to most questions. In comparison, the onset of dementia is more insidious and the patients are unaware of any cognitive difficulties. They attempt questions but are unsuccessful.[17]

Elderly depressives run a significant risk of suicide and it is rare for them to undertake such action without serious intent.[18]

It is important, therefore, to explore issues concerning self-harm.

Treatment

The management of depression in the elderly requires the use of a multidisciplinary team (psychiatrists, psychologists, community psychiatric nurses, occupational therapists and social workers). Pharmacological treatment of elderly depressives is different from that in younger adults because of the physiological changes of ageing and the co-administration of medications for physical disorders. This alters the doses at which antidepressants can be safely prescribed and, in practice, this tends to be a significant problem. The modifications of note are shown in *Table 9.3*.

Changes in elderly depressives	Effects on antidepressant treatment
Reduction in protein binding	Elevation of free drug levels
Reduced hepatic and renal function	Elevation of plasma drug levels
Increased physical illness and polypharmacy	Greater risk of adverse effects and drug interactions

Table 9.3
Effects of ageing on antidepressant treatment.

The side-effects of antidepressants are discussed in detail in **Chapter 5**, and so only those with clinical implications for older people are mentioned here. The side-effect profile of TCAs is accentuated. Effects on blood pressure and postural sensitivity may lead to frequent falls and injury. Cardiotoxicity and delirium due to high tricyclic plasma levels are more likely in those who are physically unwell. The SSRIs are generally better tolerated and so these should be first line. Of the MAOIs, moclobemide is well tolerated and seems to be particularly useful in depressed patients with cognitive impairment.[19] With most of the atypical or novel antidepressants, experience in the elderly is relatively limited. The strategies for the pharmacological treatment of depression are discussed in other chapters, and these are not necessarily different in the elderly.

ECT is often used for the treatment of depression in the elderly as it is effective and reasonably well tolerated.[20] It is often indicated in psychotic depression and is also effective in anxious or agitated elderly depressives.[21]

Psychological therapies are often used to treat elderly depressives because of their poor compliance with medication and the adverse effects of drugs. Bereavement counselling and anxiety management can be offered alone or as adjuncts to other forms of therapy. These are often indicated when, following the treatment of depression, there are specific bereavement issues that need to be addressed or there are residual anxiety symptoms. Both psychodynamic and cognitive behavioural therapies are effective in the treatment of depression in the elderly, although they are less useful if the depression is severe and has marked biological symptoms or occurs in a patient with personality disorder.[22]

Finally, family therapy merits consideration as ageing changes the role a person plays within a family and the status and privileges they afford. Depression can be a tremendous burden for those upon whom the patient is dependent, and this can lead to a wide range of feelings towards the depressed individual. These can sometimes precipitate or maintain depressive illness and so the aim of family therapy is to substitute these with more constructive feelings and means of interaction and behaviour. This is usually the task of a trained therapist.

Postpartum disorders of mood

Childbearing is a significant life event with biological and psychosocial consequences.

Physiologically, it involves many endocrinological changes and some of these have direct effects on mood. Psychologically, it involves establishing a new relationship and perhaps adjusting to a new role as parent. Socially, it may have vocational, financial and recreational implications. It is not surprising, therefore, that childbearing is associated with disorders of mood. The types of depressive disorder that occur are shown in *Table 9.4.*[23, 24]

Post-natal disorder	'Maternity blues'	Depression	Psychosis
Clinical features	Lability of mood, sadness, anxiety, crying spells, fatigue and insomnia	Depressed mood, worry about physical illness, preoccupation with somatic symptoms, insomnia, irritability, fear of harming the baby, guilt, feelings of inadequacy and loss of libido	Confusion, disorientation, irritability, anxiety, delusions and intrusive thoughts about harming the baby, emotional lability and occasionally auditory hallucinations
Usual time of onset postpartum	3–5 days	2–4 weeks	First few weeks
Frequency	50%	10–15%	0.2%
Duration of symptoms	2 days	Many months if untreated	Up to 3 months
Treatment	Self-limiting and no specific treatment indicated	Psychological therapies and physical treatment if necessary	Admission to hospital; physical treatment as necessary and supportive/psycho-logical therapies

Table 9.4
Postpartum disorders of mood.

The majority of post-natal depressive disorders are mild and transient with perhaps only a third requiring some form of treatment. Hospital management may be provided in the form of out-patient clinics or involve admission to a mother-baby unit. In-patient treatment is rare and most cases are adequately managed by GPs, community nurses and health visitors.

Treatment strategies are not necessarily different, although the means of delivery of care can be varied: in addition to those usually involved in the community, management of depression, assessments, supports and treatments may often be provided by midwives and health visitors.

Antidepressants can pass from maternal to foetal blood and into breast milk, and so their use during pregnancy and breast-feeding is associated with certain risks. Knowledge concerning these risks is limited by the fact that, if at all possible, pharmacological treatment is avoided. The known risks are summarized in **Table 9.5**.[25, 26]

Antidepressant Class	Pregnancy	Breastfeeding
TCAs	Relatively safe but avoid first trimester; stop gradually prior to parturition to avoid withdrawal in newborn	Excreted in milk; often undetectable in baby; no significant adverse effects except with doxepin
MAOIs (including moclobemide)	Risk of hypertension; risk of teratogenicity	Excreted in milk
SSRIs	Lack of sufficient data; possible link with miscarriage*	Excreted in milk; lack of data
Novel or atypical drugs	Lack of data	Lack of data

Fluoxetine

Table 9.5
Antidepressant use in pregnancy and breastfeeding.

Epilepsy and depression

Epilepsy and depressive illness are associated in a number of ways. The diagnosis of epilepsy often leads to the development of depressive symptoms because of the nature of the illness and its social stigma. Depressive symptoms can occur in the prodrome, be an ictal phenomenon, or manifest after the seizure as post-ictal depression. The latter is often severe and difficult to manage, having much in common with psychotic depression.[27] Depressive episodes between seizures are relatively common and this interictal depression is often variable in its intensity and duration with abrupt, unexpected onset and remission.[28]

The risk of suicide in an epileptic is increased five-fold, in comparison to that in the general population *(Chapter 10)*, and this is a further five-fold higher (x 25) if the epilepsy is of the temporal lobe variety (temporal lobe epilepsy — TLE).[29] The risk of deliberate self-harm is also greater in epileptics and so the development of depression is a serious concern.

The treatment of depression in an epileptic involves balancing the risk of precipitating seizures against the need to treat the depressive illness with physical measures — namely, antidepressants and ECT. All antidepressants are likely to increase the risk of seizures, either directly via effects on receptors and membranes or through pharmacokinetic interactions with anticonvulsants. TCAs tend to increase the occurrence of seizures because of their seizure-threshold lowering effect, whereas MAOIs, especially moclobemide, and SSRIs carry relatively little risk of inducing seizures.[30, 31] Clinically, the risk of an antidepressant-associated seizure can be minimized by monitoring and maintaining therapeutic blood levels of anticonvulsant medication.

In some epileptic depressives ECT may be necessary but in all cases psychological treatments should be considered, particularly when patients have considerable difficulty in adjusting to the illness. Depressive illness, in the setting of epilepsy, should be treated as necessary, accepting the fact that there may be a period during which the epilepsy is less well controlled.[32]

Personal
- Age; sex; marital status and children
- Recent stresses and social circumstances: occupation, home
- Family: relationships with parents and siblings
- Childhood: separations and losses

The attempt
- Method used
- Time of day and events prior to attempt
- Social field of the attempt: where it took place, who else was there?
- Circumstances of the attempt: details of what actually happened *(see Table 10.3)*
- Events following the attempt and attitude of others

Medical history
- Physical illness; substance abuse
- Medications prescribed

Psychiatric history
- Previous diagnosis and history of psychiatric illness
- Previous deliberate self-harm

Table 10.2
Points to consider when assessing suicidality.

followed by more direct and specific questioning: 'Have you thought about harming yourself?'

Contrary to common belief, there is no evidence that inquiring about suicidal ideation or intent prompts people to commit suicide. Often the patient appreciates that someone has understood their feelings and that they are able to share their burden. Therefore, if the possibility of self-harm is suspected, the issue must be explored.

The majority of patients who commit suicide or attempt it have seen a doctor in the weeks before. Specifically, 60–70% of suicides saw their GP in the month prior to killing themselves and half of these consultations were within a week of the event. Similarly, 50% of the psychiatric out-patient suicides saw their psychiatrist in the week before dying and, in total, a quarter of all suicides are psychiatric out-patients at the time of death.[8]

Parasuicide

The risk of suicide following parasuicide is increased one hundred-fold and 1% of parasuicides commit suicide in the first year following their initial attempt. The greatest risk is in the first six months and a significant risk remains for up to five years. One in 10 of those involved in parasuicide will eventually commit suicide and half of all suicides have a history of deliberate self-harm.

Self-poisoning is the most common method of parasuicide and is used in 90% of cases. The majority of these (75%) involve medications that have been prescribed to the patient, although paracetamol (purchased by the patient) is also very frequently used.

The prediction of suicide in an individual case is difficult. However, there are some factors of parasuicide that indicate suicidal intent and increase the liklihood of repetition. The subjective dangerousness of an attempt, carried out in isolation, with detailed planning to avoid detection, indicates its seriousness and helps to gauge the patient's suicidal intent. Frequent previous attempts in an individual with a history of violence, alcoholism or personality disorder increase the risk of further deliberate self-harm. There is also a high risk of repetition in those patients who regret having survived, continue to feel hopeless, and have no change in their circumstances as a result of the attempt.

However, it is important to note that the motivation of parasuicide attempters and those who commit suicide occasionally overlaps. Many patients fail to kill themselves, and although their intention was to die they are considered parasuicides. Conversely, some patients with the intention only to cause self-harm manage to kill themselves and are described as suicides. Hence it is necessary to distinguish those who have suicidal intent from those who have attempted suicide, perhaps to manipulate others.[6–8]

Management of suicidality

Prior to an act of deliberate self-harm

If a significant risk of suicide exists then hospital admission should be considered and compulsorily implemented if necessary. The decision as to whether the patient should be admitted depends on the degree of support available at home (family, friends or healthcare professionals) and the patient's understanding of their thoughts and ability to use supports appropriately.

Once in hospital the patient's safety should be ensured by maintaining close observation and removing potentially harmful objects, such as tablets and sharp instruments. Treatment may be started as a matter of urgency: if, for instance, there is a serious risk of suicide because of severe depressive illness, ECT may be required.

Following an act of deliberate self-harm

Following a suicide attempt, the risk of repetition is gauged by assessing suicidal intent (as above). The degree of intent at the time of the failed attempt should also be assessed, and this can be achieved by considering the points in *Table 10.3.*

Treatment

In addition to the medical treatment of any physical or psychiatric condition, social and psychological interventions should be considered. Family problems, in particular marital or relationship break-

downs, may need to be addressed by way of marital therapy or family therapy. Social support tackling employment and housing difficulties may also be required. However, for those with a history of repeated parasuicide these interventions are often of limited effectiveness.

Psychiatric illness, in particular depression, is considered a primary risk factor for suicide.[9] SSRIs are effective antidepressants that are safer in overdose than MAOIs and TCAs *(Table 10.4)* and therefore perhaps more suited to use in those patients where there is a high risk of suicide, especially as serotonin dysfunction is implicated in suicidal behaviour.[10]

The diagnosis and effective treatment of depression are known to decrease the risk of suicide and so, although the prevention of suicide is a difficult task, it is possible to some extent.[11]

- Planning and preparation involved (acquisition of tablets/implements, timing of attempt)
- Precautions (extent to which discovery was avoided, seeking a private place)
- Help-seeking behaviour (efforts following parasuicide to alert family or emergency services)
- Method of self-harm (dangerous physical methods)
- Alcohol and drugs (would attempt have been made in absence of drugs or alcohol?)
- Final act (leaving a note, saying goodbyes, putting matters in order, writing a will)

Table 10.3
Assessing suicidality.

Drug	Symptoms in overdose	Notes
MAOIs	Tachycardia, agitation, rigidity and coma	Symptoms and signs may take hours to manifest: sometimes fatal — secondary to pulmonary/cerebral oedema
Moclobemide	Disorientation/drowsiness	Safe if taken alone; can be fatal with SSRIs
TCAs	Cause arrhythmias and CNS depression; seizures can occur with some TCAs	Lofepramine is safest; TCAs often cause death, especially dothiepin and amitriptyline
SSRIs	Agitation, nausea and vomiting; seizures	Generally safe; dangerous in combination with other drugs

Table 10.4
Toxicity of antidepressants in overdose.

Key Points

- Depression is associated with stigma and disability.

- Depression can lead to a variety of psychosocial losses (relationships, education and employment).

- Depression can precipitate or exacerbate other illnesses.

- Depression is a very significant risk factor for suicide.

- Suicidality should always be assessed thoroughly (*Tables 10.2* and *10.3*) and may be an indication for in-patient hospital treatment.

References

1. Barraclough B, Bunch J, Nelson B. A hundred cases of suicide: clinical aspects. *British Journal of Psychiatry* (1974) **125**: 355–73.

2. Hawton K, Fagg J, Platt S. Factors associated with suicide after parasuicide in young people. *British Medical Journal* (1993) **306**: 1641–4.

3. Morgan G. Long term risks after attempted suicide. *British Medical Journal* (1993) **306**: 1626–7.

4. Cattell H, Jolly DJ. One hundred cases of suicide in elderly people. *British Journal of Psychiatry* (1995) **166**: 451–7.

5. Hepple J, Quinton C. One hundred cases of attempted suicide in the elderly. *British Journal of Psychiatry* (1997) **171**: 42–6.

6. Kreitman N. Suicide and parasuicide. In: Kendall RE and Zealley AK eds, *Companion to Psychiatric Studies*, 5th edn (Edinburgh: Churchill Livingstone, 1993) 743–60.

7. Kaplan HI, Sadock BJ, Grebb JA. *Synopsis of Psychiatry*, 7th edn (Baltimore MD: Williams & Wilkins, 1994).

8. Gelder M, Gath D, Mayou R. *Oxford Textbook of Psychiatry*, 2nd edn (Oxford: Oxford Medical, 1992).

9. Rihmer Z. Recognition of depression and prevention of suicide: the role of general practitioners and general physicians. *International Journal of Psychiatry in Clinical Practice* (1997) **1**: 131–4.

10. Kasper S, Schindler S, Neumeister A. Risk of suicide in depression and its implication for psychopharmacological treatment. *International Clinical Psychopharmacology* (1996) **11**: 71–9.

11. Isacsson G, Bergman U, Rich CL. Epidemiological data suggest antidepressants reduce suicide risk among depressives. *Journal of Affective Disorders* (1996) **41**: 1–8.

Index

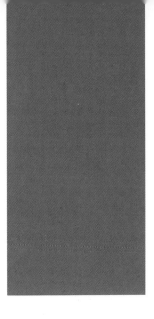